A NEW YOU
IN 21 DAYS

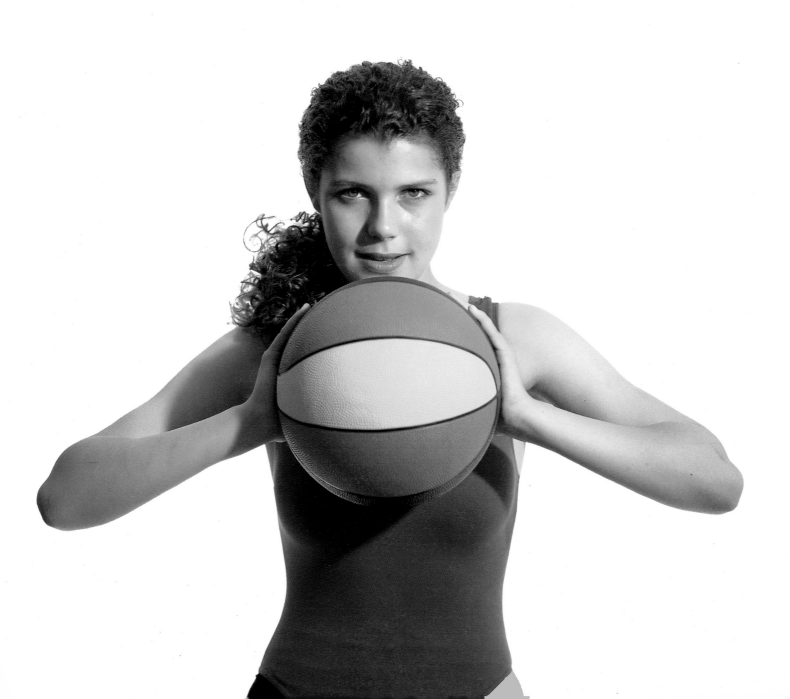

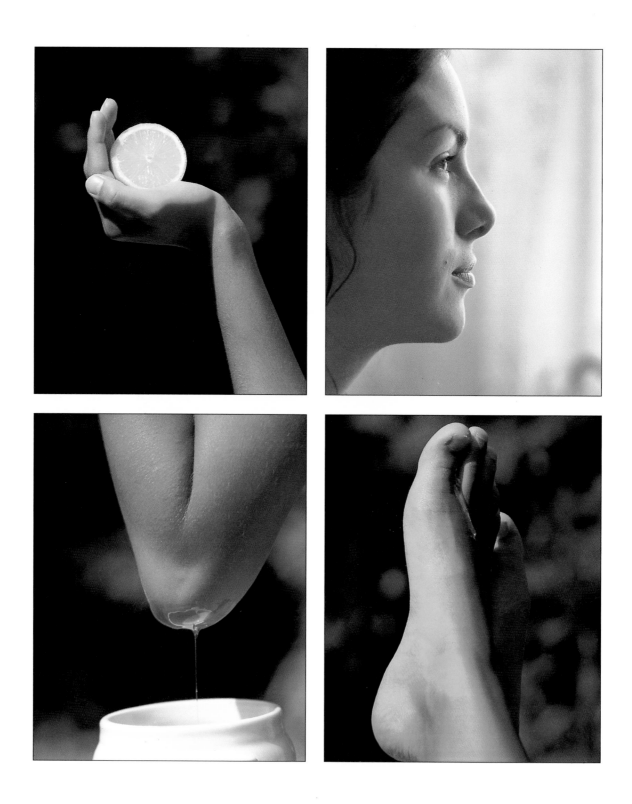

A NEW YOU
IN 21 DAYS

Kate Shapland

Special Photography by Simon Bottomley

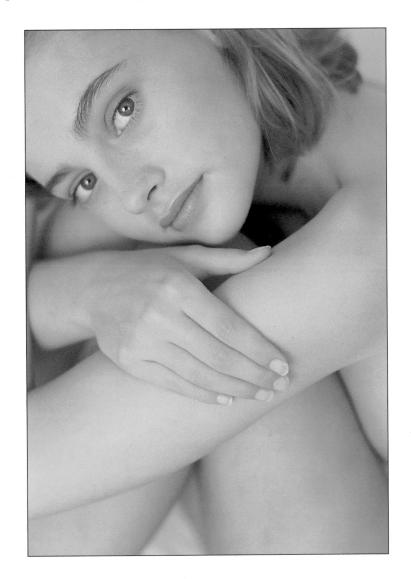

LORENZ BOOKS

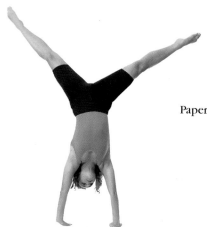

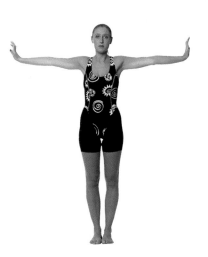

Paperback edition first published in 1998 by Lorenz Books

© Anness Publishing Limited 1995

Lorenz Books is an imprint of
Anness Publishing Limited
Hermes House
88-89 Blackfriars Road
London SE1 8HA

ISBN 1-85967-719-3

Publisher Joanna Lorenz
Project Editor Casey Horton
Copy Editors Penelope Cream, Lindsey Lowe
Consultant Dr Naomi Lewis
Designer Blackjacks

Photography Simon Bottomley
Food photography Don Last
Recipes developed by Christine France
Nutritional advisor Maggie Pannell
Exercise advisor Dean Hodgkin
Make-up Liz Kitchiner and Paul Miller from Michaeljohn
Additional make-up Bettina Graham
Models Cheryl, Jane, Joanna and Stacey

Printed and bound in Singapore by Star Standard Industries Pte. Ltd.

1 3 5 7 9 10 8 6 4 2

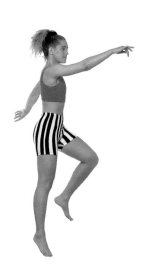

ACKNOWLEDGEMENTS
Sports clothing by Olympus, selection of plates from The Pier (retail) Ltd.
Special thanks to DB Crawford, Natasha Crittenden, Linda Fraser, Nicki Giles,
oe Henderson, Catherine McCrum, Ruth Prentice, Clare Nicholson, Nikki Reading,
RU-TEE, Lucy Shapland, Genevieve Smith, Sarah White and Sarah Beaugeard.

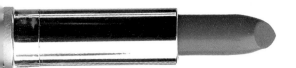
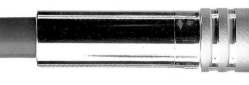

CONTENTS

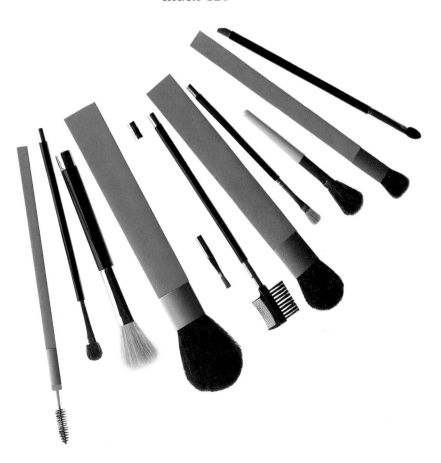

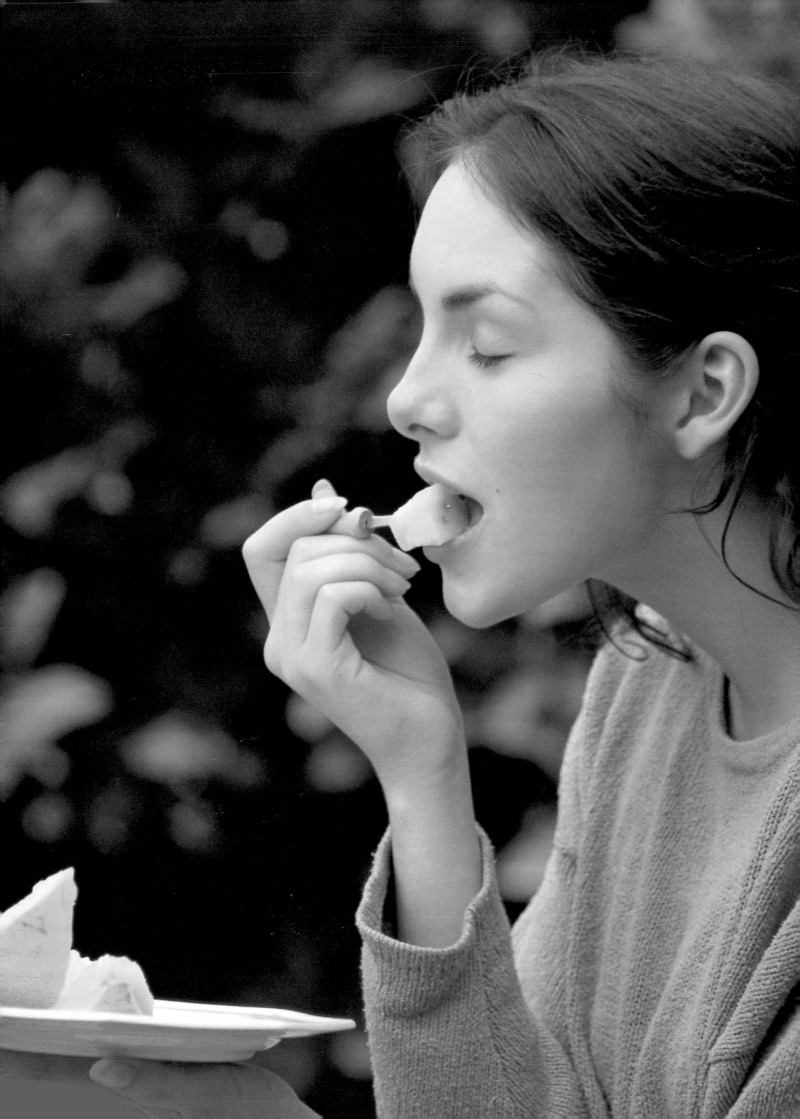

INTRODUCTION

This book is about looking better faster. In fact it's about improving your looks in 21 days; and the following pages are crammed with facts, tips, and trade secrets on achieving this through special exercise, diet, and beauty routines.

Speed is the key to successful self-improvement: achieving fast results helps to keep you inspired, because the better you look, the more confident you are and the more encouraged you will be to reach your ultimate goal. It is possible to see the sort of results in 21 days that will help you to continue eating a healthier diet, be more active and also more selfish about pampering yourself.

Depending on the goals you set yourself, you may well find that you achieve everything you have aimed for. Whatever happens, you will notice an improvement if you follow the guidelines. And when you consider how life-enhancing the results will be, three weeks is not very much time to invest in improving your shape and appearance. Good luck!

Kathy Sharpland

FIT FOR ANYTHING

ARE YOU UNFIT AND OUT OF SHAPE? YOU COULD BLAME YOUR LIFESTYLE FOR THE STATE YOU ARE IN. TODAY, EVERYTHING IS GEARED TO MAKE LIFE AS EASY AS POSSIBLE. WE DO NOT HAVE TO WALK UP STAIRS BECAUSE THERE IS USUALLY A LIFT TO CARRY US, AND WE DO NOT HAVE TO WASH CLOTHES BY HAND BECAUSE MOST OF US OWN A WASHING MACHINE TO DO THE WORK FOR US. THOSE OF US WHO ARE OFFICE WORKERS ARE AMAZINGLY INACTIVE; WE SIT ALL DAY — IN A CAR, BUS, OR TRAIN, OR AT A DESK — AND SLUMP ON A FAVOURITE CHAIR IN THE EVENING. DO YOU WANT TO IMPROVE YOUR FITNESS BUT FEEL IT WOULD BE TOO DIFFICULT? GETTING IN TRIM APPEARS TO BE HARD WORK AND TIME-CONSUMING, BUT IT DOES NOT NEED TO BE. FITNESS CAN BE ACHIEVED IN JUST THREE WEEKS. SO, IF YOU WANT A FITTER, FIRMER BODY FAST, READ ON TO DISCOVER HOW TO GET RESULTS — AND FEEL LIKE NEW — IN RECORD TIME.

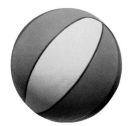

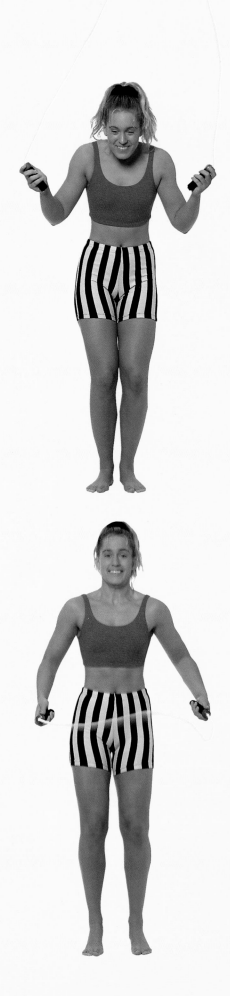

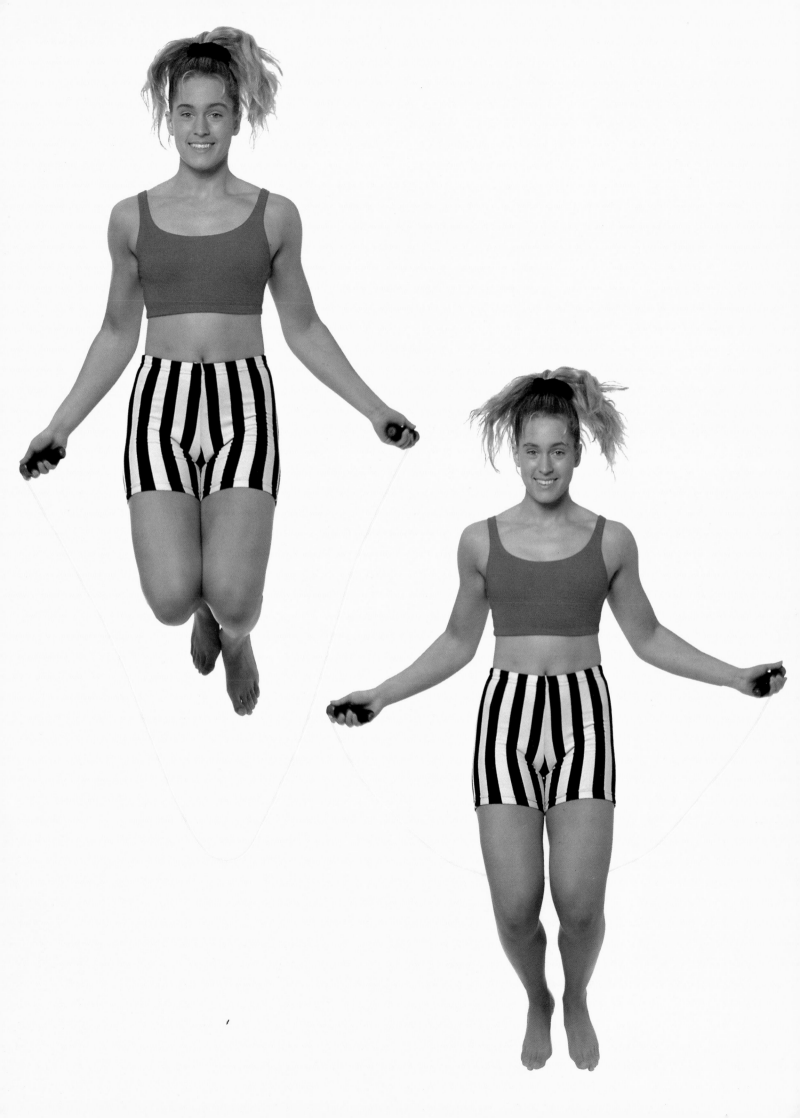

FITNESS AND EXERCISE

Fitness is the key to a healthy mind and body. It is based on stamina, strength, and suppleness – the three "S's"; better shape and self-esteem are two extra "S" bonuses. Being fit does not merely improve your physical prowess and grace, it also makes you feel better over-all. Most of us know that if we were fitter, we would have more confidence and greater zest for life. But although we are more health-conscious about our diet nowadays, regular exercise is still not a part of most people's daily lives. Surveys always draw the same conclusions as to the reasons for this: lack of time, energy, interest, and confidence. Becoming fit is neither as difficult nor as time-consuming as it may appear to be: you can get fit – and get a better body into the bargain – more quickly, easily and enjoyably than you may think.

HOW FIT DO YOU NEED TO BE?

There is no such thing as a standard fitness gauge – it all depends on your personal make-up and why you want to be fit: being robust enough to run a marathon, for example, is very different from honing the three "S's" to gain improved physical shape and health. For exercise to be of any help to you, though, it should boost your metabolism and improve your cardiovascular (heart and circulation) and respiratory (breathing) systems.

GOALS AND RECORD RESULTS

Finding a goal that will inspire you is one of the secrets of success. To achieve that goal, you must have a motive that matters enough to give you an iron will, such as improving your figure for a special event (for example, your wedding and honeymoon), buying yourself a longed-for figure-hugging dress, or simply boosting your fitness levels generally. Set the dead-

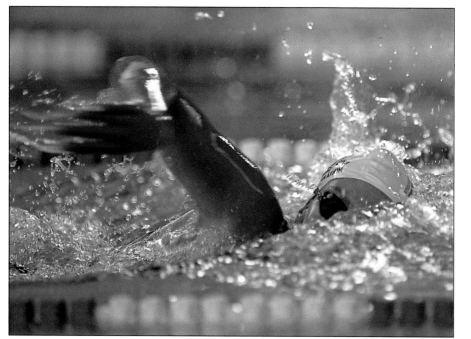

Swimming is an excellent way of keeping the whole body in good physical condition when done regularly and conscientiously.

WHY BOTHER WITH FITNESS?

Why are you reading this book? Are you fed up with having low self-confidence? Are you tired of running out of puff, being out of shape (obese, even) or always feeling under the weather? Do you often get colds, or suffer from bad pre-menstrual syndrome (PMS), stress, or sleepless nights? These are just a handful of the signs that could manifest themselves when you are unfit. So exercise is worth the effort, because when you are fitter, recurring problems such as these may ease or disappear.

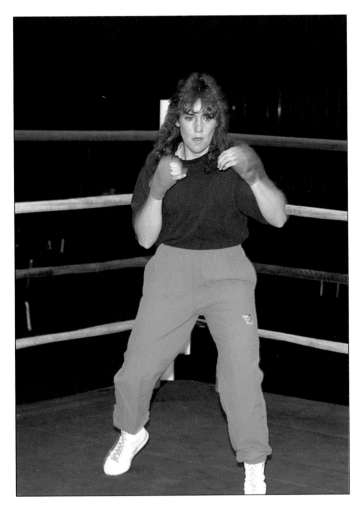

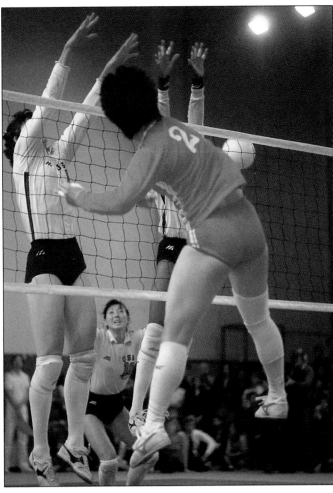

Women are increasingly attracted to strenuous sports such as boxing that until recently were considered to be solely a male preserve.

Competitive team sports such as volleyball not only provide an opportunity to improve physical fitness, they are also highly enjoyable.

line and stick to it. Depending on what you want to achieve, a three-week plan is ideal because it is not too long and if you persevere (take it week by week or day by day – whichever you find easiest), you will see results. Be realistic: if your goals are too high you are more likely to fail; if they are too low, you will not have enough of a challenge.

Goals will inspire you, but speedy results are the key to keeping up regular exercise – it is natural to want to see rewards for all your hard work – although it is advisable to build up a pattern gradually. The minimum amount of exercise you need to do to improve your personal fitness is 20 minutes 3 times a week – the "3 x 20" maxim. This means three bouts of exercise vigorous enough to make you fairly breathless (but not gasping for breath). So if you do the general fitness exercises outlined in this book 3 times a week for 20 minutes you will get fitter. If you want to see fast results, though, you need to add extra activities – such as a couple of games of tennis, swimming, or brisk walking – to your exercise quota, so that you are actually exercising six days a week.

Taking part in a team sport once a week is a good idea: not only will it make you fitter, slimmer, and happier, the competitive spirit will

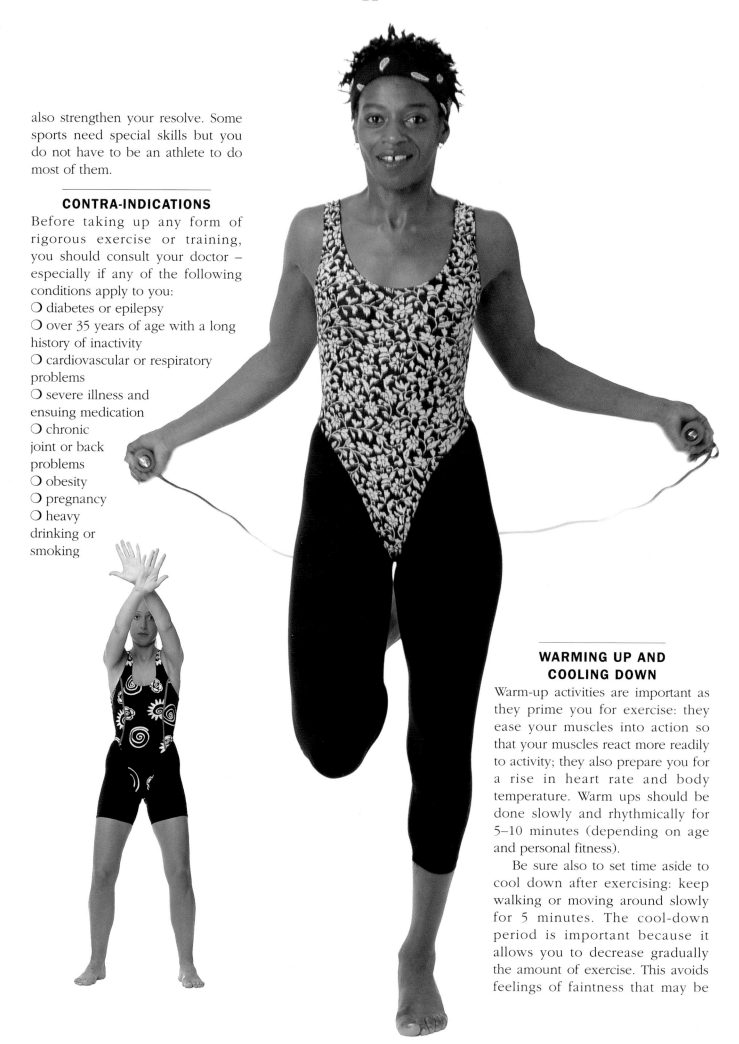

also strengthen your resolve. Some sports need special skills but you do not have to be an athlete to do most of them.

CONTRA-INDICATIONS

Before taking up any form of rigorous exercise or training, you should consult your doctor – especially if any of the following conditions apply to you:

○ diabetes or epilepsy
○ over 35 years of age with a long history of inactivity
○ cardiovascular or respiratory problems
○ severe illness and ensuing medication
○ chronic joint or back problems
○ obesity
○ pregnancy
○ heavy drinking or smoking

WARMING UP AND COOLING DOWN

Warm-up activities are important as they prime you for exercise: they ease your muscles into action so that your muscles react more readily to activity; they also prepare you for a rise in heart rate and body temperature. Warm ups should be done slowly and rhythmically for 5–10 minutes (depending on age and personal fitness).

Be sure also to set time aside to cool down after exercising: keep walking or moving around slowly for 5 minutes. The cool-down period is important because it allows you to decrease gradually the amount of exercise. This avoids feelings of faintness that may be caused by the pooling of blood below the waist that occurs during vigorous exercise.

YOUR PULSE RATE

Monitoring your pulse rate allows you to keep a check on whether you are exercising adequately. The maximum heart rate for an adult is roughly 220 beats per minute minus your age in years. The ideal heart rate during exercise is in a target zone of 65-80 per cent of this figure. The aim of exercise is to get your heart rate to within a certain range. These are the ideal exercise heart rate ranges for the different ages:

Age	Pulse Range
20+	130–160
30+	124–152
40+	117–144

To find out your active pulse rate per minute, rest two fingers lightly on your pulse immediately after exercising, count the beats for 10 seconds and multiply by 6.

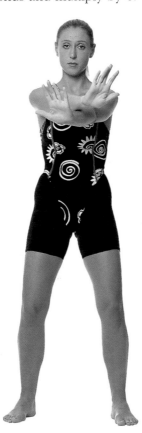

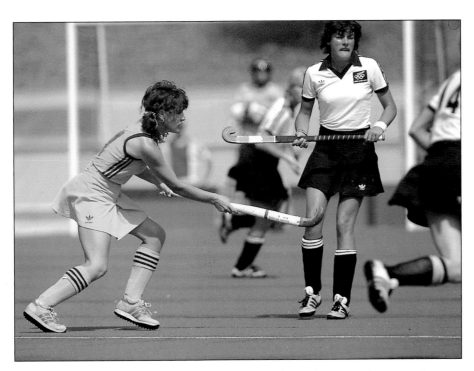

Hockey is a demanding sport that strengthens the legs, is beneficial to the heart and lungs, and significantly improves co-ordination.

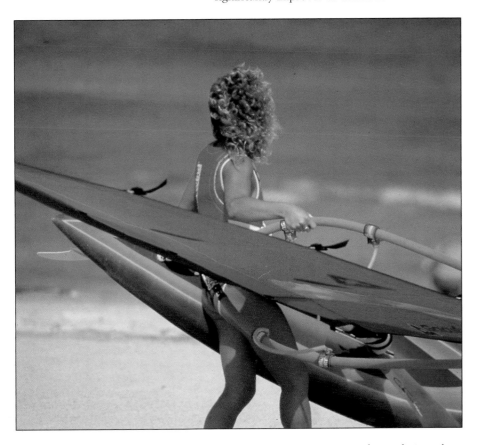

A good many water sports demand strength, stamina, and a fine sense of balance. Wind surfing is no exception to the rule.

EXERCISES FOR GENERAL FITNESS

This exercise routine helps to improve over-all fitness and should take you roughly 30 minutes to complete. Aim to do it three times a week and try to do extra aerobic exercise – such as swimming, walking or cycling – on the other days (aerobic exercises include any activity that can be done rhythmically and continually and that boosts the efficient uptake of oxygen). To warm up your muscles before exercising, either spend two minutes running up and down the stairs, walking briskly, cycling, or doing the special warm-up exercises outlined below.

Think of warm-up exercises as a way of easing your body into increased activity. The movements should be slow and rhythmical, not sharp and jerky.

WARM-UP EXERCISES

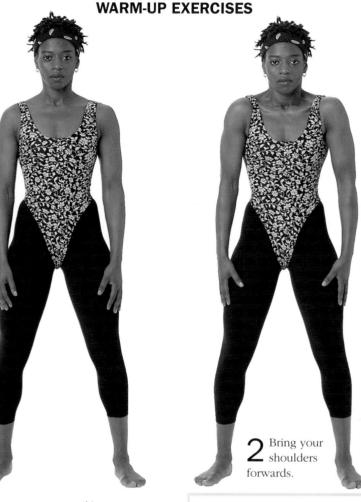

Warm-up Exercise A

1 Stand upright with your feet apart and in line with your shoulders, with your arms hanging loosely at your sides and your shoulders down.

2 Bring your shoulders forwards.

IMPORTANT NOTE

If you feel any pain – or experience anything other than the normal sensation of muscle fatigue – stop exercising. Quit if you feel dizzy too. Always work out at your own pace; and skip exercise if you are ill, have a virus or a raised temperature.

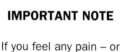
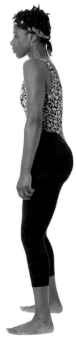
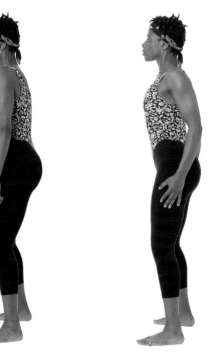

3 Then raise them as high as you can.

4 Now move your shoulders back as far as possible. Finally, bring them back to the start position.

REPETITION GUIDE FOR GENERAL FITNESS EXERCISES

Toning Exercises	Repeats/Time Allowance
Warm-ups	5 minutes
Press-ups	10 repeats
Lying Flies	10 repeats
Reverse Curls	10 repeats
Sit-ups	10 repeats
Squats	10 repeats
Cool Downs	3–5 minutes
Aerobic Exercise	20–30 minutes

The recommended 10 repeats are for beginners – you should aim to repeat each exercise (from Warm-ups to Cool Downs) 15 times, or as often as is comfortable. Start by doing this set of exercises twice a week, work up to three times a week and combine it with some other form of exercise – ideally aerobics – for the time suggested above.

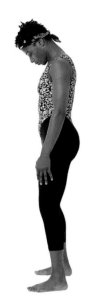
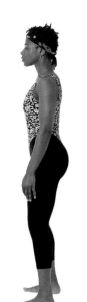
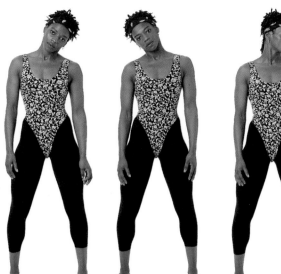
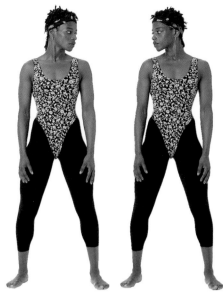

Warm-up Exercise B

1 Maintain an upright posture as in Exercise A. Tip your head forwards so that your chin is almost resting on your chest.

2 Raise your head, stretching and lengthening your neck as you return to the upright position. Repeat 4 times.

3 Now tip your head to the left, keeping your shoulders down. Bring it back to the centre and then stretch and lengthen your neck.

4 Repeat Step 3 but tip your head to the right side. Repeat 4 times on each side, remembering not to raise your shoulders.

5 Keep your head upright and turn so that you are looking over your left shoulder. Then face forwards again and stretch and lengthen your neck.

6 Now turn and look over your right shoulder. Face forwards again and stretch and lengthen your neck. Repeat Steps 5 and 6 four times, then do the whole sequence again twice.

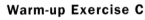

Warm-up Exercise C

1 Stand with your feet fairly wide apart; lean forwards slightly from your hips keeping your chest lifted and back straight.

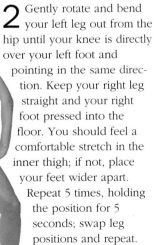

2 Gently rotate and bend your left leg out from the hip until your knee is directly over your left foot and pointing in the same direction. Keep your right leg straight and your right foot pressed into the floor. You should feel a comfortable stretch in the inner thigh; if not, place your feet wider apart. Repeat 5 times, holding the position for 5 seconds; swap leg positions and repeat.

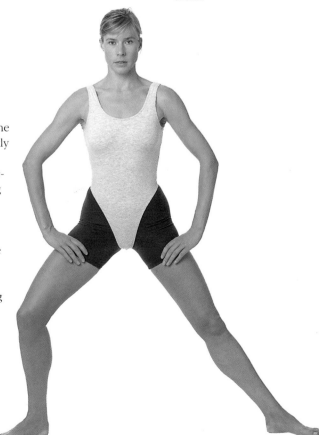

THE GENERAL EXERCISES

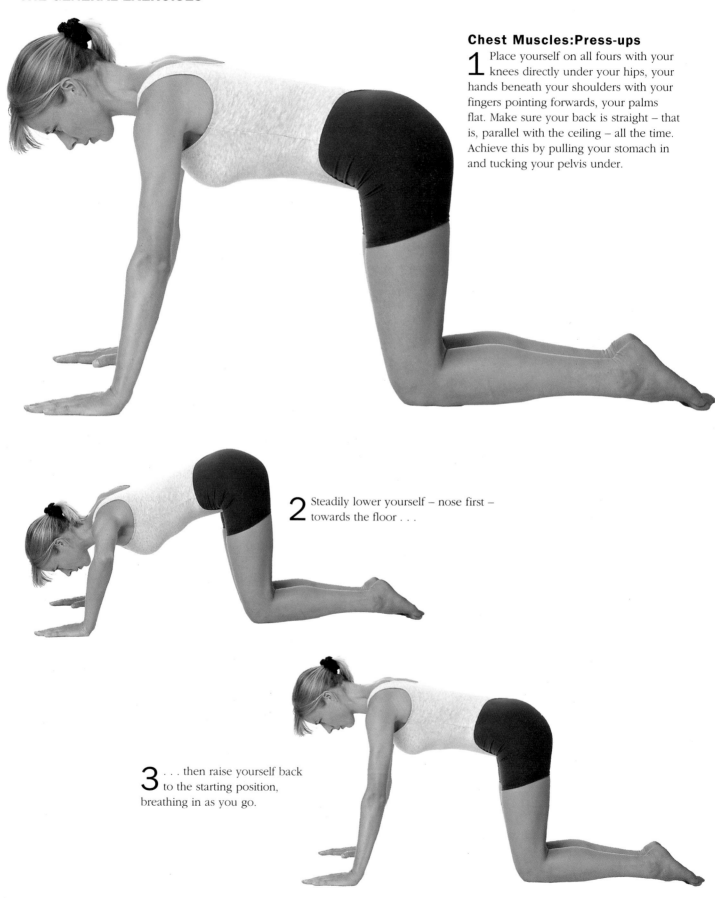

Chest Muscles:Press-ups

1 Place yourself on all fours with your knees directly under your hips, your hands beneath your shoulders with your fingers pointing forwards, your palms flat. Make sure your back is straight – that is, parallel with the ceiling – all the time. Achieve this by pulling your stomach in and tucking your pelvis under.

2 Steadily lower yourself – nose first – towards the floor . . .

3 . . . then raise yourself back to the starting position, breathing in as you go.

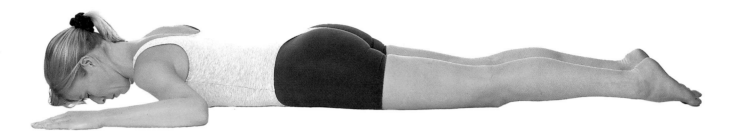

Upper Back Muscles:Lying Flies

1 Lie on your front on the floor with your hips down, and keep your body relaxed. Rest your forehead on the floor, your arms out on each side at right angles to your body, elbows bent.

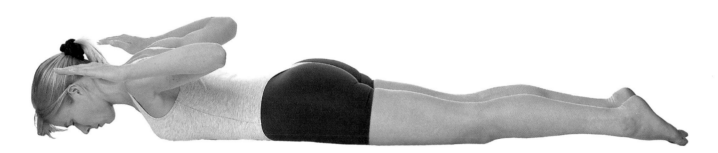

2 Keeping your elbow bent, steadily lift both arms, making sure they are parallel to the floor.

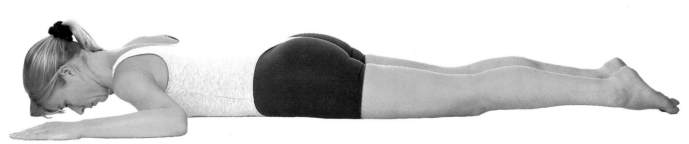

3 Lower your arms once again. Make sure you don't pull your elbows back; keep them in line with your shoulders and keep your hips and feet in contact with the floor all the time.

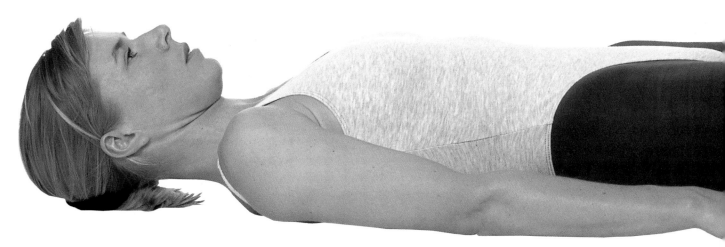

ABDOMINAL MUSCLES

When you do these exercises, keep your lower back pressed into the floor throughout and work slowly, with total control. In the Upper Abdominals exercise, lift your head and shoulders as one unit, never separately; roll up from the top of your head; imagine you are holding a peach between your chin and your chest and keep this gap constant throughout. Make sure your face muscles are relaxed all the time.

Lower Abdominals:Reverse Curls

1 Lie flat on your back on the floor, arms by your sides, palms flat on the floor beside you.

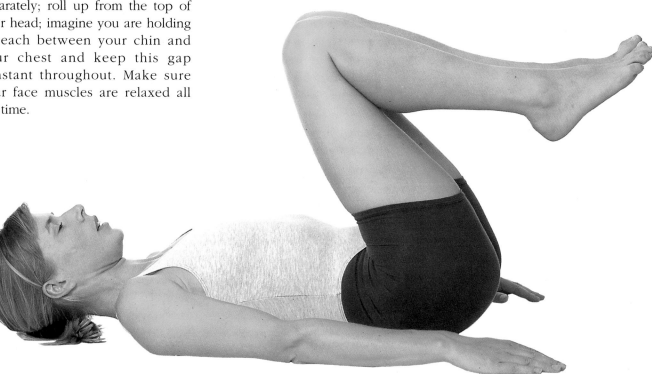

2 While keeping your arms and hands flat on the floor, bring your knees in towards your chest one at a time, and once there, keep both knees together in the bent position.

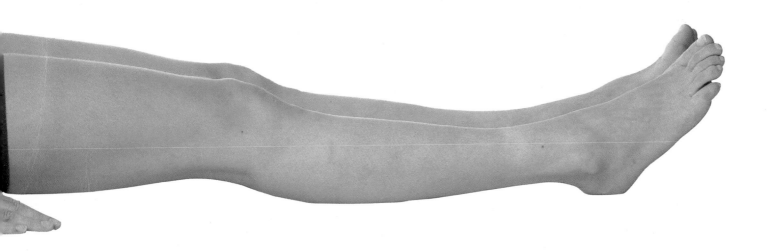

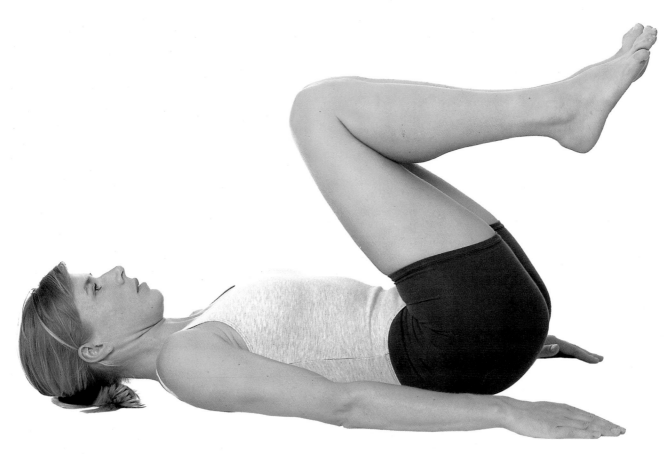

3 Breathe in and, keeping your spine firmly pressed into the floor, pull in your abdominal muscles while at the same time curling up your coxyx (tail bone) to bring your knees closer to your chest. Keep your feet relaxed throughout. Lower your body to the starting position, exhaling as you go down.

Upper Abdominals:Sit Ups

1 Lying flat on the floor with your arms by your side, palms flat on the floor, bend your knees and keep your feet flat on the floor a little distance apart in line with your hips.

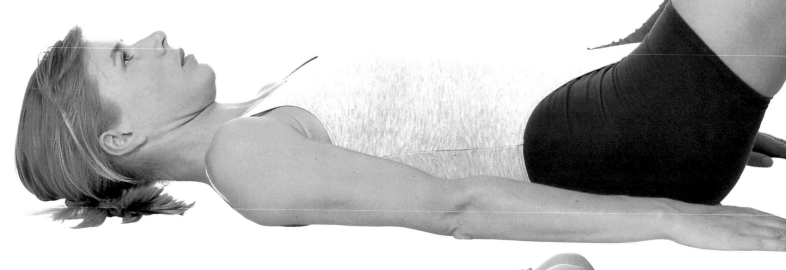

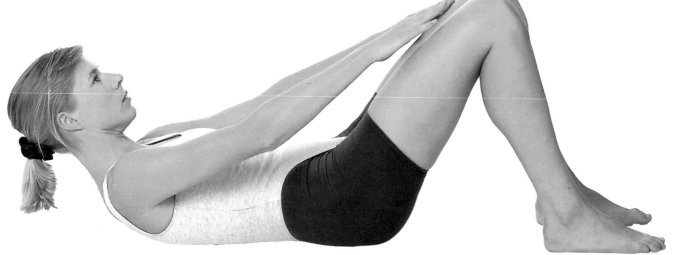

2 Lift your head and shoulders – inhaling as you move up – and push your fingertips towards your knees keeping your arms straight.

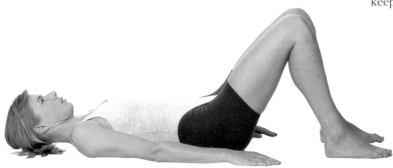

3 Lower your body back to the starting position, exhaling as you go down; repeat the movement.

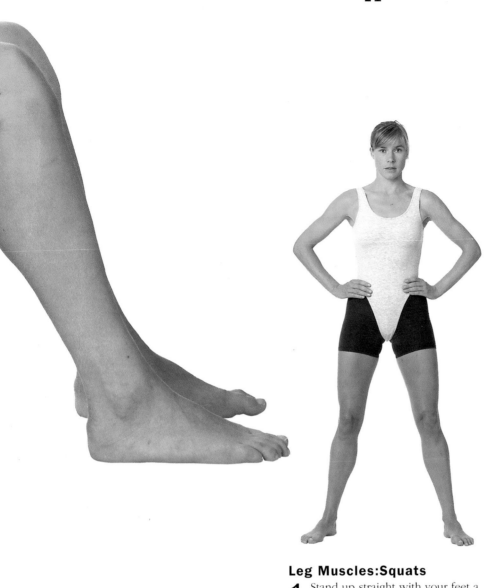

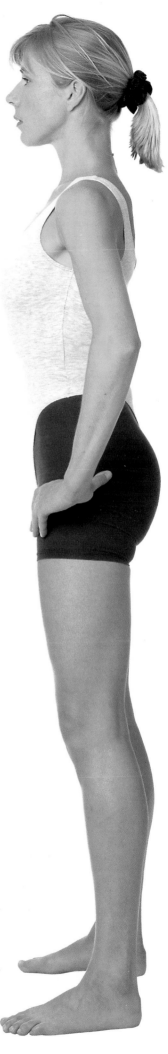

Leg Muscles:Squats

1 Stand up straight with your feet a little wider than shoulder-width apart. If you stand on tiptoe, this exercise tones your calf muscles and your quadriceps, the muscles on the front of your thighs; if you angle your toes slightly outwards while on tiptoe, it benefits your inner thighs.

2 Resting your hands on the front of your thighs and keeping your arms straight, steadily bend your legs to a squatting position, exhaling as you go down.

3 Then, inhale as you rise steadily back to the starting position. When you do this exercise, it is important to keep your back straight and your knees flexible. Don't let your knees bend further forward than your toes.

SPORTS ACTIVITIES

Team sports and work-outs at the gym are not only fun, they also give you the chance to add to your exercise quota for the week, and therefore reach your self-improvement goals that much faster. The benefits of taking part in specific sports and of working out are given here.

Badminton: aerobic; improves joint flexibility, stamina, leg and shoulder tone and strength; 30-40 minutes continuous play burns up around 200-800 calories.

Golf: improves arm, shoulder and leg tone, and strength (you walk four to five miles when you do a round of golf).

Jogging: aerobic; improves stamina, leg strength and tone; an hour's jogging burns up 200-350 calories. If you think that jogging or running will suit your new active way of life, take the standard precautions before you start: check with your doctor and, as with all aerobic exercise, increase the pace gradually; always wear the right trainers (and support bandages if your joints are weak).

DIETING COMBINED WITH EXERCISE

You will lose weight if you limit your food intake, but not as quickly or as evenly as you would if you combined a balanced weight-loss diet with regular exercise. Exercise increases your metabolism, and, if you want to lose weight more quickly, you need to exercise in conjunction with dieting.

MAKE EXERCISE EASY TO DO

Your body cannot "store" fitness, so once you have started, you have to keep exercising regularly. Make your routine flexible: if you think it is going to be hard to maintain, don't choose an activity that requires good weather or a long detour from your office or home.

Tennis: aerobic; boosts stamina and suppleness; strengthens and tones your shoulders, forearms, calves and thighs; play energetically (ideally twice a week) for an hour and you will burn up around 300-400 calories.

Brisk walking: aerobic; strengthens and tones your legs.

Cycling: aerobic; builds stamina; tones your legs.

Skipping: aerobic; boosts stamina, strength and leg tone. Start by doing 3 skipping sets for 30 seconds a time with a 5-minute

---

HOUSEWORK TIME NEEDED TO BURN UP 100 CALORIES:

○ Ironing: 50 minutes
○ Sweeping the floor: 30 minutes
○ Washing-up: 28 minutes
○ Vacuuming: 40 minutes
○ Polishing furniture: 52 minutes

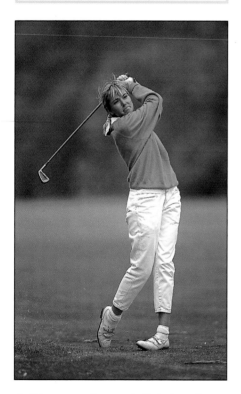

Golf is a sport that particularly benefits shoulders, arms, and legs. Playing a round involves a good deal of walking.

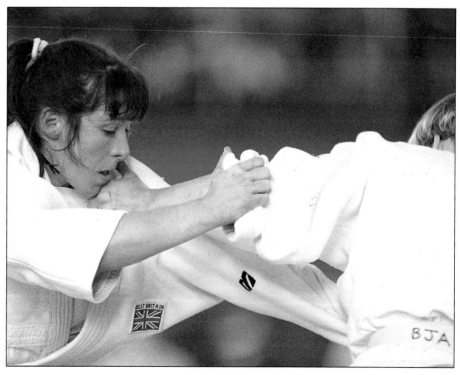

Judo is a body contact sport and one of the major martial arts. It requires a good deal of strength, agility, and physical courage.

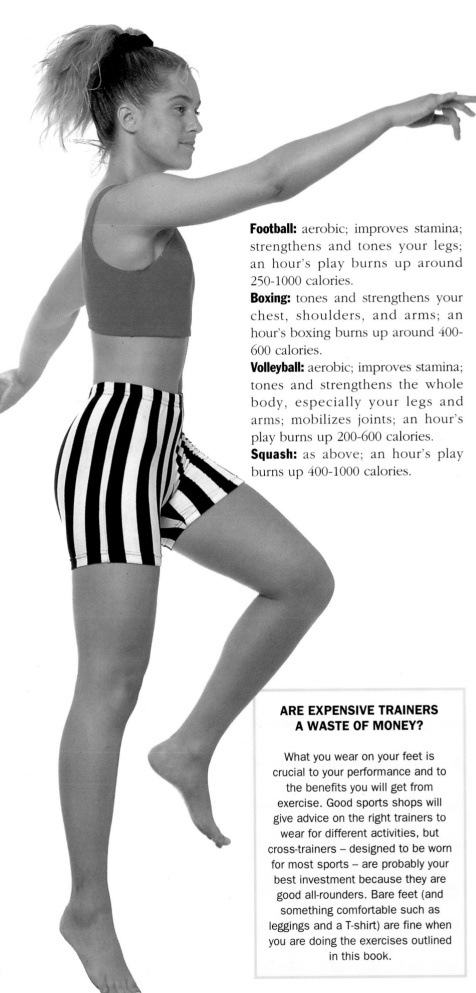

GYM-BASED BENEFITS

Aerobics: specific aerobics classes combine exercise with constant movement for up to an hour; they are fast fat-burners and an ideal activity to do regularly if you are after speedy results.

Circuit, cross, resistance, or weight training: aerobic; increase stamina, strength and suppleness; an hour of circuit training burns up between 350-550 calories.

Step classes: aerobic; improves stamina; tones and strengthens your lower torso (bottom, thighs and calves); an hour-long class burns up between 500-800 calories.

Yoga: improves posture; tones, strengthens, and relaxes the body; loosens joints; an hour of yoga burns up about 200 calories.

break after each set; build up to skipping for 2 minutes with a 10-minute break and also increase the repetitions.

Rebounding: aerobic; bounding on a mini trampoline is a fun way to get fit at home.

Swimming: aerobic; swimming is one of the fastest (and best) ways to boost overall fitness, muscle tone, joint flexibility, and relaxation. Do 4 lengths of a 25 m/25 yard pool, rest for a minute and build endurance by reducing rest time and increasing swim time; within a fortnight you will be noticeably fitter and firmer; an hour's breaststroke burns between 500-800 calories.

HELP FOR PMS

Exercise is the last thing you feel like doing when you are pre-menstrual. But if you do push your-self now, you will feel more relaxed and relieve the symptoms. If you cannot face an aerobics class, go for a swim: this will ease pre-menstrual cramp and put you in a better mood.

Football: aerobic; improves stamina; strengthens and tones your legs; an hour's play burns up around 250-1000 calories.

Boxing: tones and strengthens your chest, shoulders, and arms; an hour's boxing burns up around 400-600 calories.

Volleyball: aerobic; improves stamina; tones and strengthens the whole body, especially your legs and arms; mobilizes joints; an hour's play burns up 200-600 calories.

Squash: as above; an hour's play burns up 400-1000 calories.

ARE EXPENSIVE TRAINERS A WASTE OF MONEY?

What you wear on your feet is crucial to your performance and to the benefits you will get from exercise. Good sports shops will give advice on the right trainers to wear for different activities, but cross-trainers – designed to be worn for most sports – are probably your best investment because they are good all-rounders. Bare feet (and something comfortable such as leggings and a T-shirt) are fine when you are doing the exercises outlined in this book.

BODY SHAPE

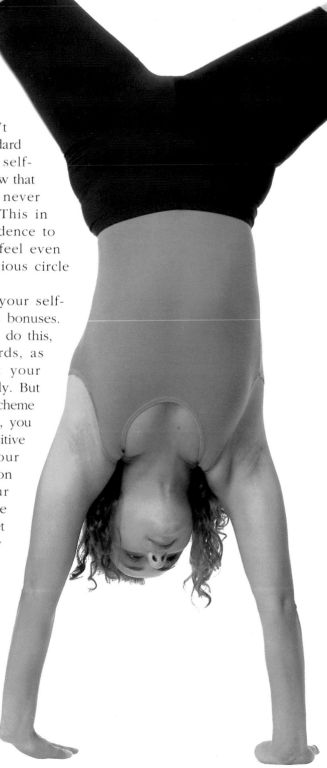

The shape of your body is unique; it is important to remember this because the basic skeletal and muscular form that you inherit is unchangeable. Features such as your height, foot size, shoulder width and the length and shape of your legs, nose, fingers and toes combine to produce a whole. Each person is an individual, with characteristics particular to their genetic make-up.

BODY BRACKETS

Although we come in a variety of shapes and sizes, the human body is cast from three basic moulds. Often, features from two or three of these body types are jumbled with our individual characteristics, but it is the more dominant features that slot us into one of the following groups: ectomorphs; mesomorphs, and endomorphs.

Ectomorphs are usually small- and slender-framed with long limbs, narrow shoulders, hips and joints. They have little muscle or body fat. Mesomorphs have medium to large – but compact – frames with broader shoulders, pelvic girdle and well-developed muscles. Endo-morphs are naturally curvaceous, with more body fat than muscle, wider hips, shorter limbs and a lower centre of gravity than the other two body types.

SELF-IMAGE

If you are a bit on the tubby side, it can be annoying to hear someone who you think is poker-thin whining about being overweight. But there is a logic behind this that stems from self-image. Very few of us actually see ourselves as we really are. We tend to misjudge our bodies with sweeping claims to fatness, even when we have only a spot of excess flab around our midriff to show for it. And although

it sounds amazing, the way we behave in every-day life (and think others see us) often tallies with our self-image. It's a vicious circle: we think that we don't measure up to the standard beauty ideal so our self-esteem dips, often so low that we feel that we will never have a better body. This in turn causes self-confidence to plummet further, we feel even worse, and so the vicious circle continues.

Taking control of your self-image brings enormous bonuses. And the faster you can do this, the greater the rewards, as speedy results boost your confidence more quickly. But before you undertake a scheme to get into better shape, you must work on your positive thinking: realize your potential by deciding on (and accepting) your body model, then use this as your goal. Forget conventional beauty ideals – you don't have to have mile-long legs to have a dynamite figure; what you already have – your basic shape – is great. It just needs per-fecting, and that is something that everyone can do.

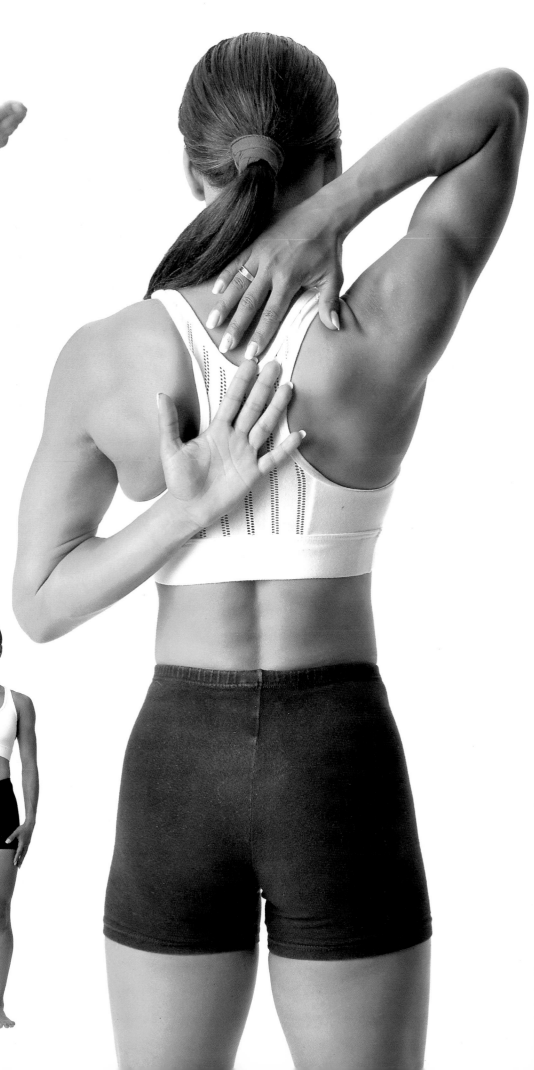

GOOD POSTURE

Even though it sounds like some pointless exercise from your schooldays, there is real wisdom in the old dictum "head up, shoulders back, bottom in". The difference that good posture makes to the look of our bodies is enormous, mainly because when we are standing properly our abdominal muscles are in their correct supporting role and the whole body is aligned so it looks leaner and taller. Good posture is also helpful to our mental and physical health; some alternative therapies (such as the Alexander Technique) are based on the principle of correct posture because it can ease back pain, stress, and even headaches.

Posture Exercise Stand in front of a mirror, try these exercises and see what they do for the shape of your body:

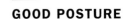

1 Do this exercise facing yourself first, then turn so you are sideways on:
○ Lift your head up and lengthen your spine.
○ Tuck in your chin and your bottom.
○ Bring your shoulders back and down.

2 Now stand with your legs slightly apart.
○ Check whether your weight is evenly spread.
○ Keep your shoulders and hips level and your weight balanced between the heel and ball of each foot.

TROUBLE SPOTS

Very few people are able to say honestly that they are totally happy with their body. Everyone has at least one gripe – if it is not big feet, it is thin hair or knobbly knees. All these perceived "flaws" can be improved or disguised, but as anyone who has ever tried (and failed) to move the fat that sits on strategic points such as hips, thighs, stomachs, and buttocks knows, it is much easier to hide the flaws than to tackle them. Trouble spots such as these are notoriously stubborn to shift, but it is possible to alter your outline with a combination of diet and exercise.

COMMON PROBLEMS

Any of the following can be discouraging, but remember – each problem has a solution.

Slack stomachs Our stomachs become flabby when the abdominal muscles slacken; this usually happens through lack of exercise. Your abdomen extends from just under the bustline to the groin, and

The best way to assess your figure is to stand in front of a full-length mirror. Be honest with yourself, and look for areas that need improving.

FINDING AND IMPROVING YOUR TRUE FORM

Step 1: Confront Your Body
Go on, be brave. Strip to your underwear, stand in front of a mirror and have a good look at your body. Take your time and be tough but realistic. You may have disliked your thighs since you were 16 – and they will probably never be those of a supermodel – but if you look hard enough you might just find that they are not as bad as you have always thought they were, and that improving them is not going to be that hard after all.

Step 2: Put Your Complaints In Writing
Note down all the things that irk you (and that you can do something about) as well as those that you like or do not mind. Then go through your list of dislikes, ticking the things that you really want to do something about. Also, make a mental note to start appreciating your good points: the more you focus on them the less you will notice the not-so-good zones.

Step 3: Action Checklist
Now, add a set of action points under the problem zones you have listed. If you want to firm up your arms for that sleeveless sundress you have been unable to wear for a decade of summers, make notes like this:
Flabby Upper Arms
❍ Do Basic Exercises.
❍ Check Diet.
❍ Exfoliate/Moisturize.
Finally, add your goal(s) and your deadline to the top of the list and put it somewhere where you are going to see it frequently.

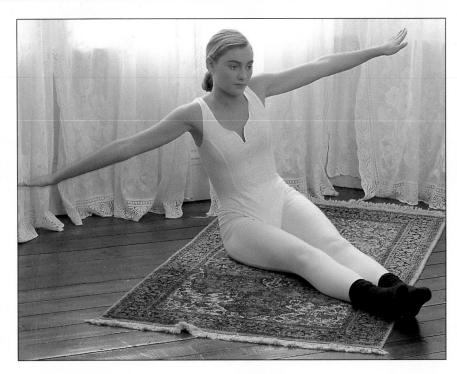

TWO QUICK THIGH-TONERS

If you do not have time to do a full exercise routine, grab 10 minutes in the morning and evening to warm up and do these two exercises.

○ **Outer Thighs:** sit on the floor with your legs straight out in front and hold your arms out to the sides as shown left. Roll sideways on to your bottom – go right over on to your outer thigh and then roll right over on to the other thigh. Do this 20 times.

○ **Inner Thighs:** stand upright and consciously tighten – and hold – your buttock muscles for a slow count of five. Repeat with your thigh muscles and then your calf muscles. You can do this while you are waiting for your bath to run, standing at the bus stop, and so on.

it is packed with muscles that criss-cross to form a wall to hold the abdominal contents in place – a bit like a corset. Exercise is not the only way to keep your stomach flat though: weight is also an important factor and the long-term answer is diet and exercise.

Thunder thighs Thighs – like bottoms and busts – are a great source of discontent, whether it is because they are too flabby, muscular, or skinny. You inherit the basic shape of your thighs, but that does not necessarily mean that you were born with the excess fat that may now be covering them. Thigh size and tone can certainly be altered with the right diet, correct body care and regular exercise. Sports such as cycling, skiing, tennis, squash, and riding (a great inner-muscle firmer) will tone your thighs, as will weight training for specific areas of the body.

Large bottoms There are three large muscles in our buttocks: *gluteus maximus, medius,* and *minimus.*

These create the shape, but not the size, of our rear ends. It is the tone of these muscles and the fatty tissue around them that gives us the bottoms we have. The good news is that buttock muscles respond well to exercise, which means that any

effort you put into bottom-toning exercises will be rewarded quite quickly. Locomotive exercises – such as fast walking, running upstairs, and jogging – are especially good bottom trimmers. Other exercises are given in the Basic Exercise Routines.

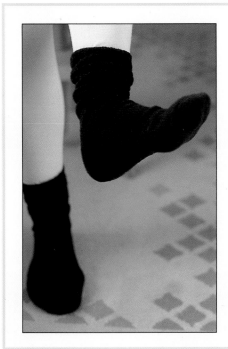

ANKLE EXERCISES

Whenever you remember – while sitting at your desk or relaxing in the evening – move your ankles around in a clockwise motion 10 times, then repeat anti-clockwise.

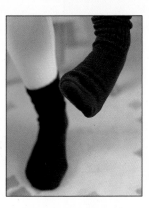

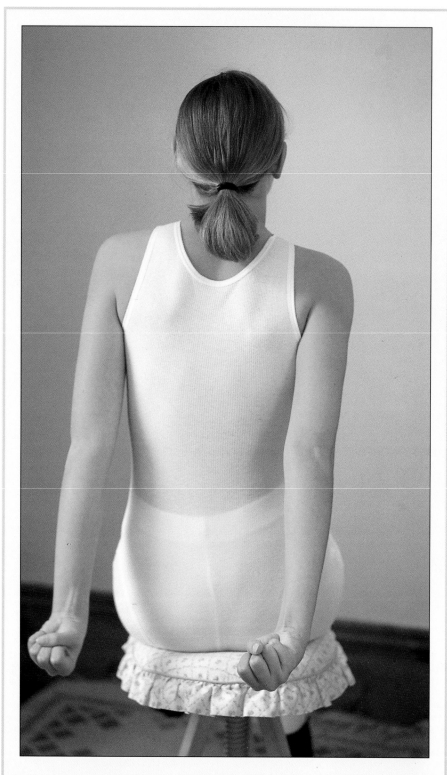

FLABBY ARM FIXER

To firm up flabby arms, add this exercise to your daily exercise routine, or spend five minutes doing it twice a day. Sit on a chair holding your hands in loose fists, and, with your arms extended out behind, make downwards punching movements backwards and forwards.

Slack upper arms Our arms do not really change shape much during our lives, unless we lose or gain a lot of weight. Muscle tone is the main problem, but, as in the case of thighs, exercise and specific weight training will tone up and re-shape flabby arms; very often, any changes in body shape that happen through exercise and diet are noticeable most quickly on your upper arms.

Droopy breasts Breast shape and size only really change when our weight swings dramatically, or during pregnancy, breast-feeding, menstruation, or if taking oral contraceptives. Gravity is the bust's worst enemy, especially if the breasts are not given proper support, because it literally drags the breasts down and slackens their tone. Although the breasts are supported by suspensory ligaments, they do not contain any muscle (the milk glands are buffered by protective fatty tissue) so you cannot noticeably reverse lost tone. However, if you exercise the pectoral muscles beneath your armpits you will give your breasts a firmer base and more uplift.

Thick ankles Trim and slender ankles that seem set to snap with every step are a great asset. But if you are not blessed with these, or if your ankles tend to become stiff and puffy from fluid retention, you need to master the art of deception and brush up on some ankle improving exercises.

Assess the flexibility of your ankles by sitting on a chair or stool with your feet on the floor and, while keeping your heel down pull the rest of your foot up as far as it will go: if the distance between your foot and the floor measures 12-15 cm/5-6 in your joint flexibility is good; if it is between 10-12 cm/ 4-5 in it is fair; and if it is less than that, your joint flexibility is poor.

The following exercises will help to improve the muscles that support your breasts.

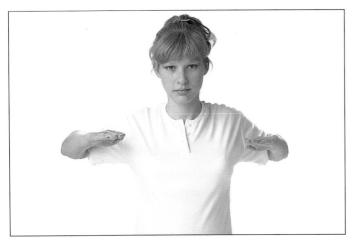

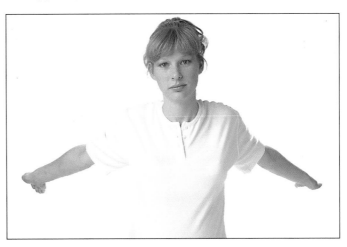

1 Stand erect and bend your arms at the elbows, holding your arms horizontally in front of your chest, with your fingertips touching. Move your elbows back as far as they will go, with a firm, quick movement. Remember to keep your lower arms level, as shown. Return to the starting position and repeat as many times as you wish.

2 Resume the position you took in Step 1, but this time, as you move your elbows back, straighten your arms, so that you fling them behind you. Repeat several times.

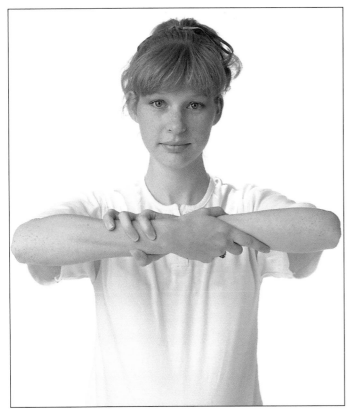

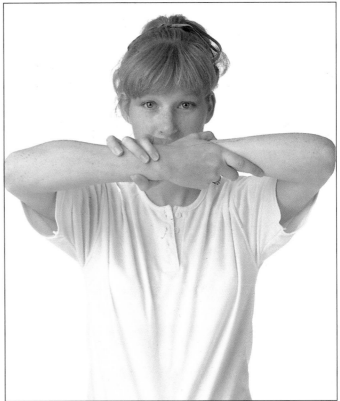

3 Stand erect and hold your arms in front of your chest, with elbows bent. Grasp your left arm just above the wrist with your right hand, and your right arm just above the wrist with your left hand, as shown. Now pull on each arm, as if you were trying to pull your hands apart, but maintain a tight grip. Hold for a few seconds. Relax your hands and then repeat again several times.

4 Now raise your arms and hold them out in front of your mouth; repeat Step 3 in this higher position. If you wish, you can also do the exercise holding your arms out just in front of your waistline.

BASIC EXERCISE ROUTINE

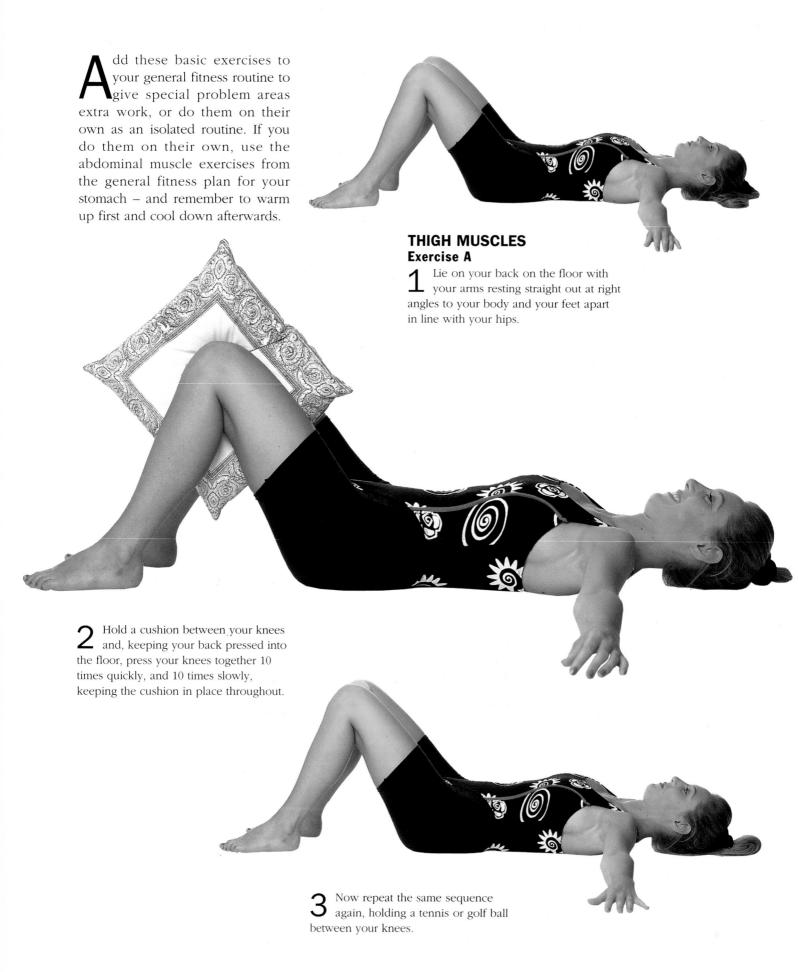

A dd these basic exercises to your general fitness routine to give special problem areas extra work, or do them on their own as an isolated routine. If you do them on their own, use the abdominal muscle exercises from the general fitness plan for your stomach – and remember to warm up first and cool down afterwards.

THIGH MUSCLES
Exercise A

1 Lie on your back on the floor with your arms resting straight out at right angles to your body and your feet apart in line with your hips.

2 Hold a cushion between your knees and, keeping your back pressed into the floor, press your knees together 10 times quickly, and 10 times slowly, keeping the cushion in place throughout.

3 Now repeat the same sequence again, holding a tennis or golf ball between your knees.

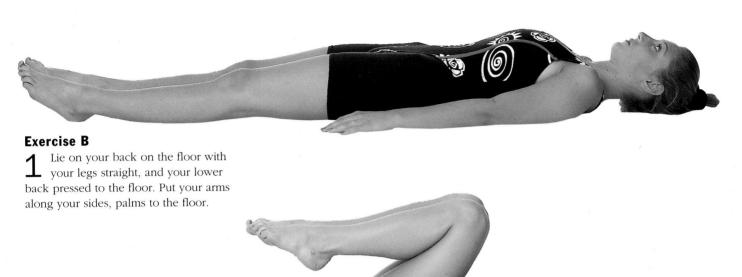

Exercise B

1 Lie on your back on the floor with your legs straight, and your lower back pressed to the floor. Put your arms along your sides, palms to the floor.

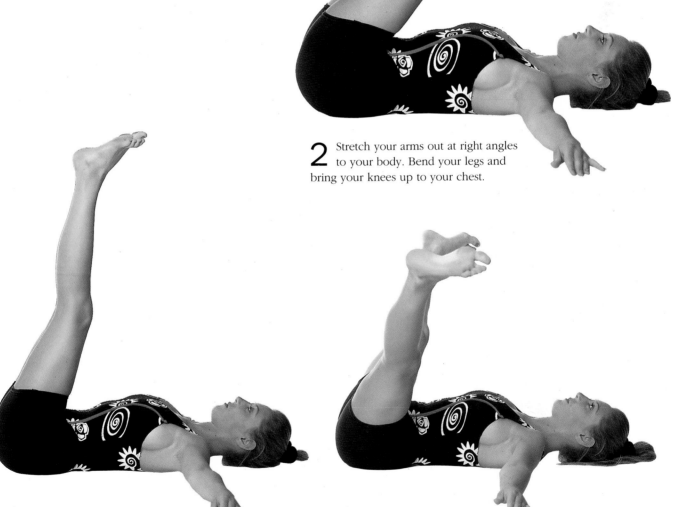

2 Stretch your arms out at right angles to your body. Bend your legs and bring your knees up to your chest.

3 Keeping your legs together, steadily straighten them so that they are pointing up towards the ceiling. Keep your feet relaxed.

4 Slowly open your legs out sideways – as wide as you can – then close them again. Repeat the exercise (Steps 2-4) 4 times. When you get used to the exercise, you can do it with small weights tied to your ankles.

Exercise C

1 Stand sideways on to a chair or table (lightly holding the edge to maintain your balance) with your shoulders down and relaxed, and with your knees bent and your feet facing forwards.

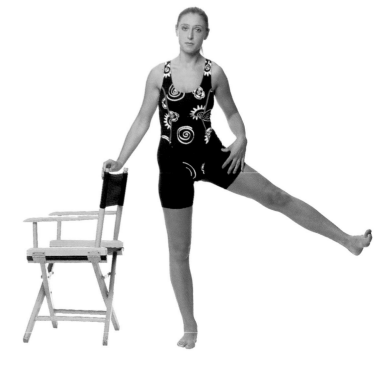

2 Lift your left hip slightly and slowly move your leg out and up (no higher than 45 degrees), keeping your foot and knee facing forwards. Make sure you do not let your body tilt – keep it as straight as possible. Carefully lower your leg. Repeat the whole exercise 10 times, then turn and repeat with the other leg.

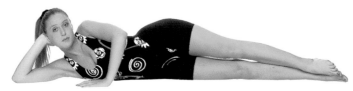

Exercise D

1 Lie on your right side on the floor with your legs out straight. Support your head with your right hand.

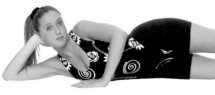

2 Bend your lower leg behind you to maintain balance and tilt your hips slightly towards the floor; your head, hips, knees, and feet should all be facing forwards. Balance yourself with your left hand on the floor in front of you.

3 Slowly lift your upper leg, then bring it down to touch the lower one; raise it again and repeat this action 6 times. Turn over and repeat Steps 1-3 on the other side.

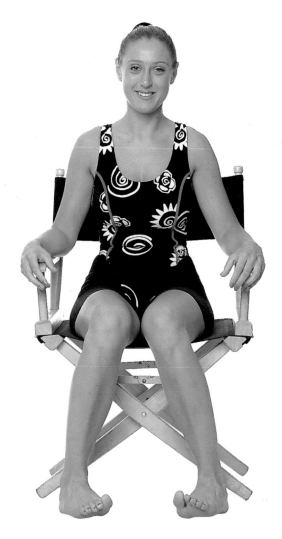 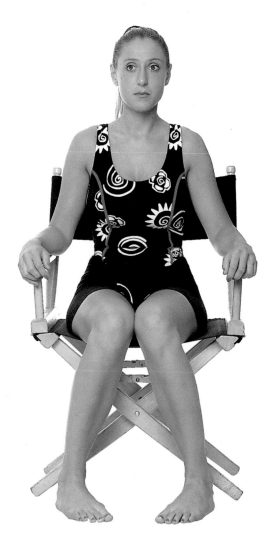

ANKLES AND CALF MUSCLES
Exercise A

1 Sit up straight on a chair, with your knees together and heels on the floor and slightly apart, in line with your hips. Bring your big toes up (as high off the floor as possible) and roll your feet in towards each other.

2 Now tilt and move both feet down and outwards from the ankle, keeping your big toes raised as much as possible as you roll your feet on to their outer edges. Repeat 10 times.

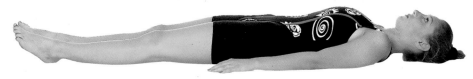

Exercise B

1 Lie flat on your back on the floor with your legs straight.

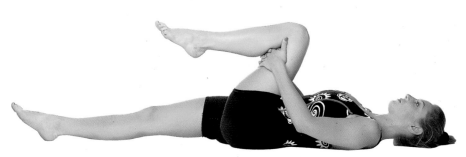

2 Bring one leg up and hold it beneath the back of your thigh so that it is pulled towards your chest. Rotate your foot 10 times in a clockwise direction and 10 times anti-clockwise. Repeat with the other leg. Increase the number of repeats to 20 for each foot, working alternately in groups of 7.

BUTTOCK MUSCLES
Exercise A

1 Stand upright and lightly hold the back of a chair or the edge of a table with both hands to maintain your balance. Put your weight on your right leg and turn your left leg out from the hip.

2 Keeping your foot flexed, take your left leg back as far as you can without bending it at the knee, forcing the movement or over-arching your back. Repeat with the other leg. Repeat 5 times for each leg and gradually build up to 20 repetitions.

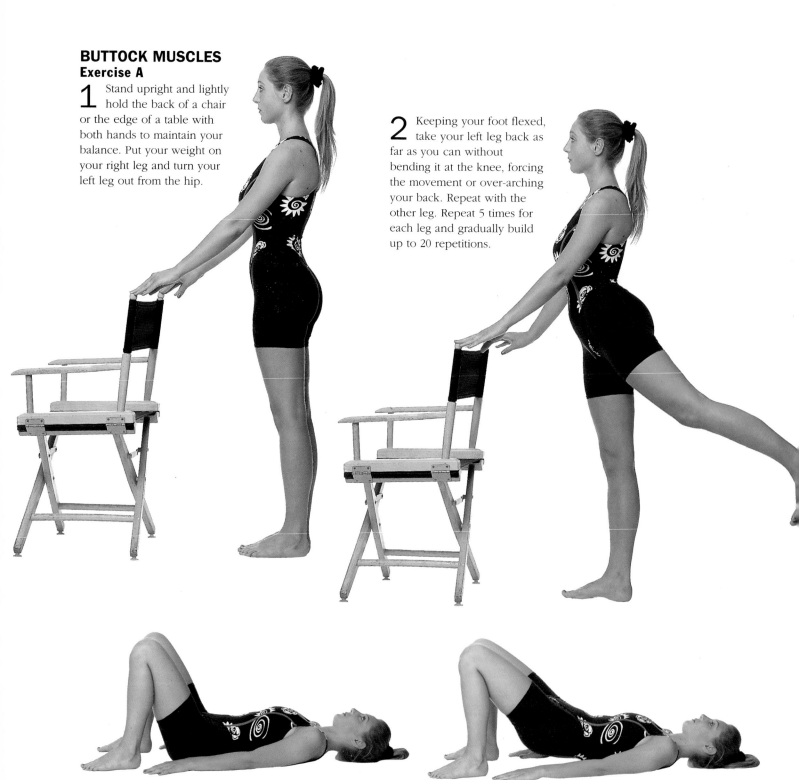

Exercise B

1 Lie on your back with your knees bent and your feet slightly apart, in line with your hips. Place your arms by your sides, palms flat on the floor.

2 Place your weight on your shoulders and upper back (not your neck), raise your bottom to a comfortable height and tighten your buttock muscles, keeping your feet flat on the floor and your arms by your sides. Hold for several seconds. Lower your bottom to the floor. Repeat 5 times, building up to 20 repetitions.

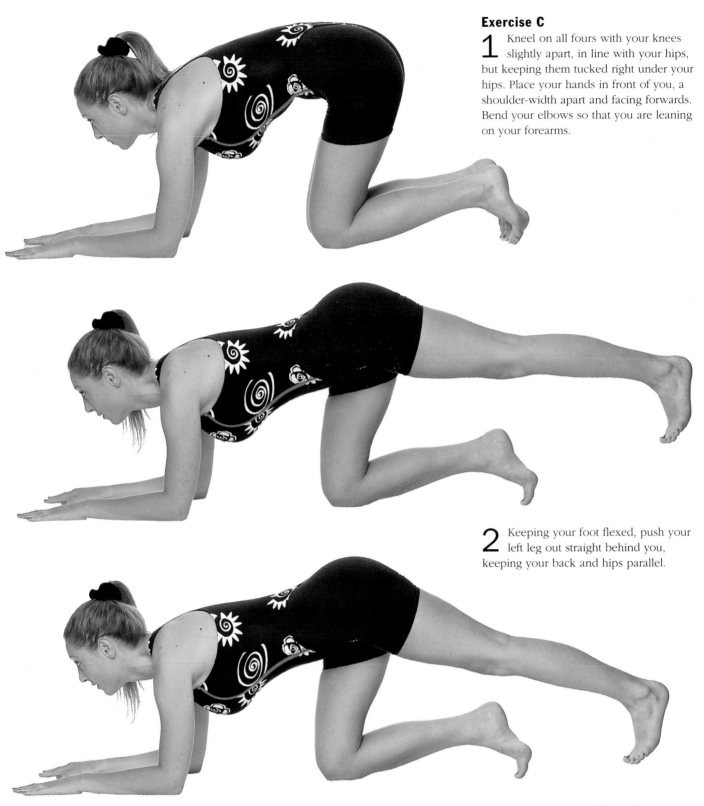

Exercise C

1 Kneel on all fours with your knees slightly apart, in line with your hips, but keeping them tucked right under your hips. Place your hands in front of you, a shoulder-width apart and facing forwards. Bend your elbows so that you are leaning on your forearms.

2 Keeping your foot flexed, push your left leg out straight behind you, keeping your back and hips parallel.

3 Bring your leg and foot down to the floor, keeping your foot flexed and your leg straight. Repeat Steps 2 and 3 twelve times. Return to the original position, then repeat the exercise with your other leg. Build up to 20 repetitions.

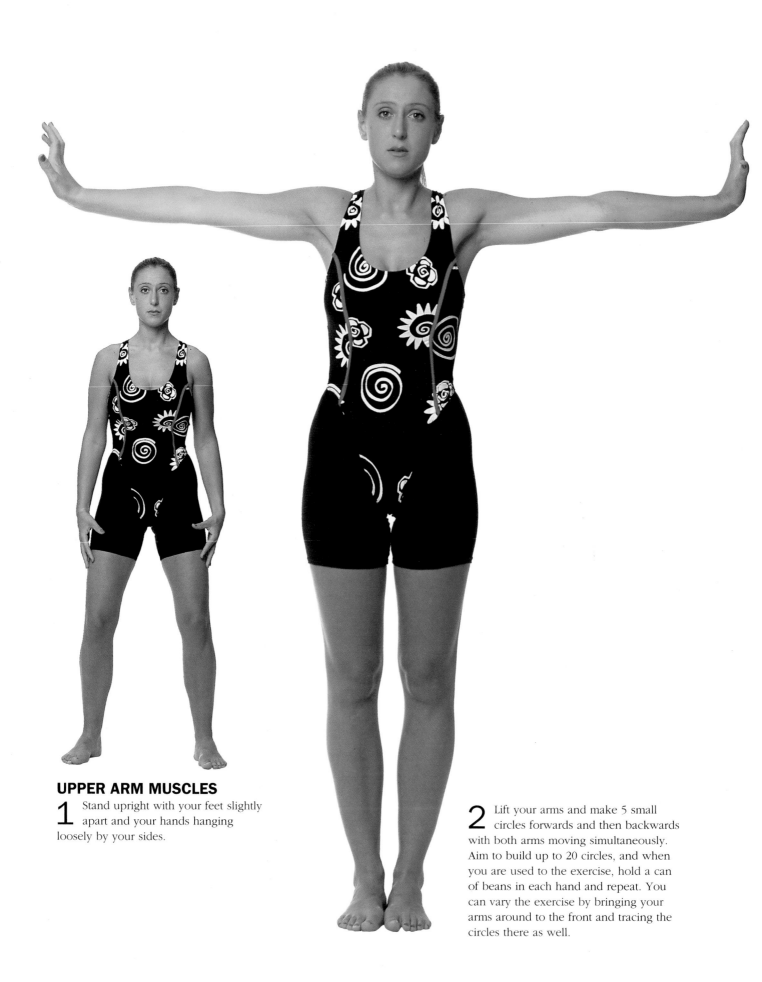

UPPER ARM MUSCLES

1 Stand upright with your feet slightly apart and your hands hanging loosely by your sides.

2 Lift your arms and make 5 small circles forwards and then backwards with both arms moving simultaneously. Aim to build up to 20 circles, and when you are used to the exercise, hold a can of beans in each hand and repeat. You can vary the exercise by bringing your arms around to the front and tracing the circles there as well.

BUST (PECTORAL) MUSCLES
Exercise A

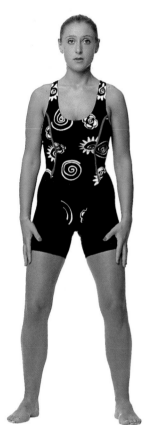

1 Stand upright with your feet slightly apart in line with your shoulders. Keep your shoulders up, your back straight, and your bottom and stomach tucked in. Keep your legs slightly bent. Let your arms hang loosely by your sides.

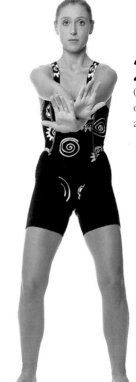

2 Make a scissor movement across the front of your body (at waist-level) by crossing one hand over the other while holding your arms straight out in front.

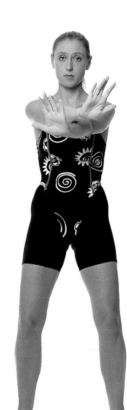

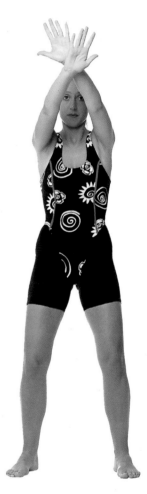

3 Raise your arms to chest level and repeat the action.

4 Then repeat the action holding your arms at head level. Keep the scissor movements controlled as you swing; do 20 repetitions at each level.

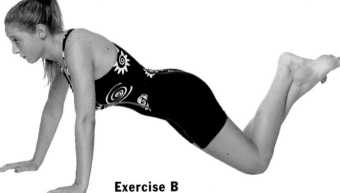

Exercise B

1 Kneel on all fours as if you are about to do press-ups, with your legs raised at the back and your feet crossed. Your arms should be straight.

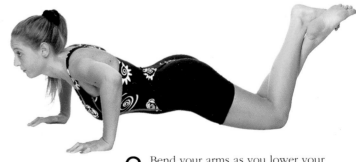

2 Bend your arms as you lower your body to the floor. Do this 10 times to begin with, and build up to 30 repetitions.

EXERCISE AND STRESS

We push ourselves at such a cracking pace these days that feeling stressed can, at times, almost become the normal way to feel. A bit of stress is quite useful because it helps to keep us on the ball, but being under prolonged pressure, and ignoring physical signs such as shaky hands, hyperventilation, and a fast heartbeat is not at all healthy. So if any of these sensations sound familiar to you, resolve to make time every day to relax your body and free your mind of problems.

DAILY RELAXATION TECHNIQUE

❍ Lie flat on the floor and shut your eyes. Take a deep breath and exhale twice, then breathe normally.
❍ Slacken your feet: let them go floppy, then relax your ankles, knees and thighs.
❍ Push your tummy out as far as you can, hold it there and then relax it completely, letting it move in and out freely while you breathe easily.
❍ Relax your shoulders, and then feel them drop back to the floor.
❍ Relax your facial muscles completely, then move the focus to your mind: force yourself to clear it – blank out and forget the day's problems – and enjoy emptying your head. All you should be thinking about now is whether your body is completely at ease; if you become aware of a tense muscle in your body, release it.
❍ Rest like this – blissfully relaxed – for a minimum of 10 minutes; when you have had enough, open your eyes and get up slowly.

HOW EXERCISE HELPS YOU TO RELAX

Exercise does not just tone your muscles, it also eases the muscular aches and pains that go hand-in-hand with stress; it also distracts your mind from the worries that make you tense. Regular exercise – and especially yoga – lifts your mood (remember how good you felt the last time you did some invigorating exercise?) and soothes your mind. As you become fitter, you will find that your ability to cope with mundane problems that crop up improves.

YOGA – A GOOD ROUTE TO RELAXATION

Yoga is an exercise technique and ancient doctrine based on achieving mind, body, and spiritual harmony. The belief is that when all these elements are in tune with each other, mental and physical health is at a peak. As well as improving

INSTANT RELAXATION

Stand by an open window and take deep, steady breaths for a slow count of 10 or 12. Then hold your breath for about 10 seconds, releasing it with a long, low "aaah". (Do not try this more than twice or it might make you feel a bit dizzy or faint.)

joint mobility, suppleness, shape and self-image, yoga can dispel the headaches and tiredness brought on by stress and nervous tension. The practice involves many active principles, but the most popular ones that are used in Western teaching are as follows.
❍ **Asana, or postures:** These are held for several minutes at a time and, together with the correct breathing, perfected to give certain physical, spiritual, and emotional benefits before each new step is learned.
❍ **Pranayama:** This is deep, slow breathing which is done while sitting – either in a lotus position, or on a chair that allows your spine to stay straight.
❍ **Relaxation:** Up to 15 minutes is spent resting (usually lying flat on

Right: Complete relaxation is fundamental to yoga teaching
Opposite: Two yoga asanas.

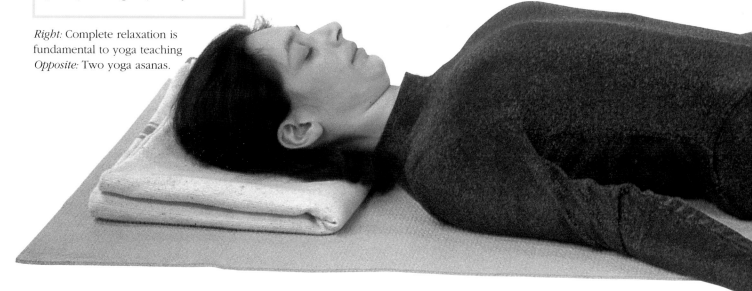

the floor) after yoga to help your mind and body unwind and recharge. Yoga principles and postures are best learned with a teacher, rather than out of a book.

NECK AND SHOULDERS – TENSION FOCUS

Anyone who has ever been tied to their desk or hunched over a computer keyboard or typewriter for long periods without a break knows all about the discomfort that a stiff neck, back, and shoulder "knots" can cause. Our upper torso is usually the focal point for mental and physical stress, and the stiffness this causes can lead to headaches and back pain. One of the best ways to avoid and relieve this type of physical stress is to get up and walk around the room regularly, stretching and loosening your shoulders by circling them backwards and forwards as you go.

IMPROVING YOUR RESPIRATORY AWARENESS

Our emotional state is reflected by our breathing patterns. When we are under strain or nervous, we tend to either hyperventilate (over-breath) or inhale short, shallow breaths – a habit that you can only break when your attention is drawn to it. Take stock and examine the way you are breathing now: is your breathing pattern regular and steady? If not, take a couple of deep breaths and start again, this time making a conscious effort to breathe steady, equal, calm breaths.

RELAXATION CHECKLIST

If you find yourself becoming tense, grab 10 minutes at the end of each day to run through this progressive relaxation checklist.

❍ Check your body: tense every little bit of it, then consciously relax every part. Bunch your toes, then free them; clench your thigh and buttock muscles, then let them relax; pull in your stomach muscles and let them go; hunch your shoulders, then relax them; clench and relax your hands several times.

❍ Check your breathing pattern: inhale deeply and slowly, hold your breath for a couple of seconds, then release it again, letting your body flop as you exhale.

❍ Check your posture: sitting, standing and walking badly can also produce knots and tightness in the muscles in your back, neck, and shoulders.

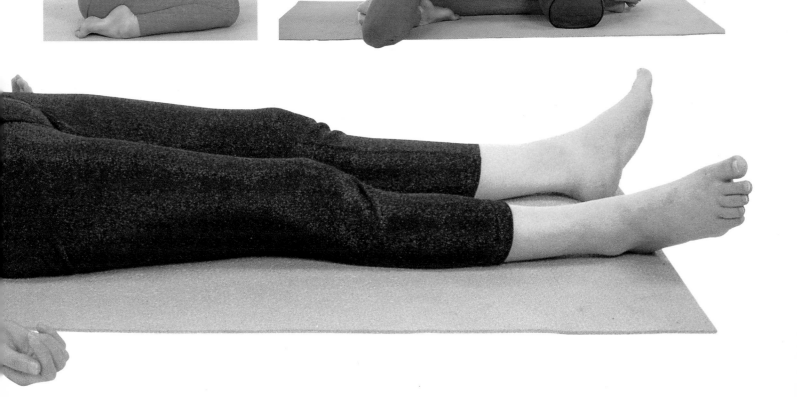

FACIAL EXERCISES: A QUICK FRESHENER AND TONER

Tension shows in your face when your features look drawn and your expressions frozen and rather set. A good laugh is the best way to relax a tense face, but this exercise routine also helps to liberate and tone the key muscles quickly; try it when you are sitting in the bath – not at the traffic lights.

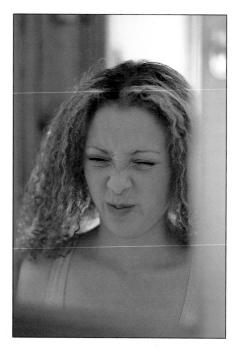

1 Scrunch up your whole face for a few seconds so that your nose is wrinkled, your forehead furrowed, and your eyes and mouth are tightly closed.

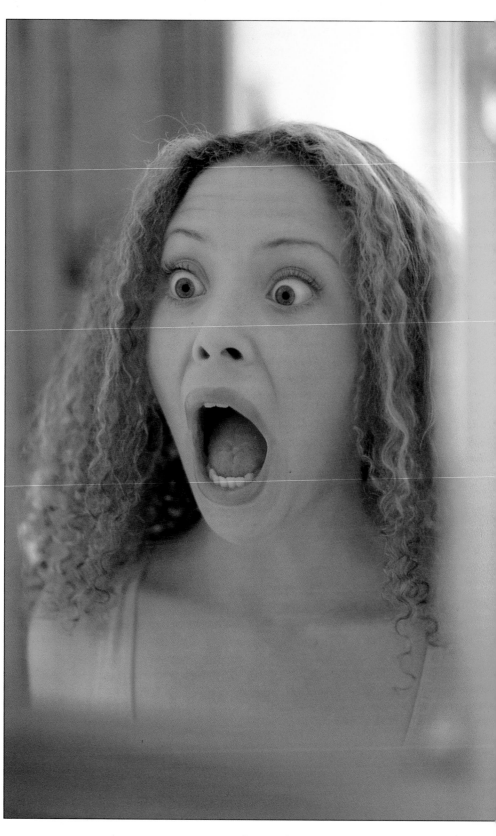

2 Do the opposite: open your mouth and eyes as wide as you can (as if you are silently screaming) to release your throat muscles.

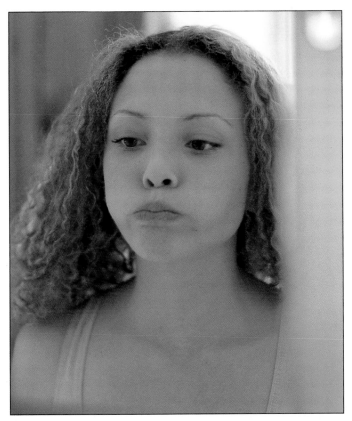

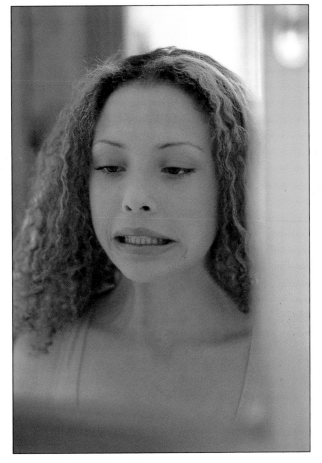

3 Close your mouth again, purse your lips, and push your mouth up to the left, then to the right.

4 Grin – as if from ear to ear – and open your eyes wide again.

5 Hold and repeat the grin, but this time, tuck in your chin to tighten your neck muscles.

EXERCISES FOR RELAXATION

As well as helping your body to relax by reducing muscle tension, these stretch exercises can be done to increase flexibility or to ease muscles, or cool down after exercising. Ease your body into these stretches: you should not be jumping or bouncing around, and the exercises are not supposed to be uncomfortable. Remember to breathe slowly and rhythmically too. The positions should be held for at least 10 seconds, but if you want to increase your flexibility, stretch the major muscle groups for a minimum of 30 seconds.

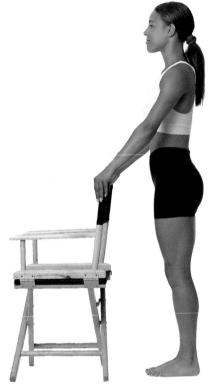

FRONT OF THIGHS

1 Stand upright with your hands on the back of a chair.

2 Bend your left leg up behind your body and clasp your ankle with your left hand. If you can't reach far enough, put a towel around your foot (not your ankle) and hold each end of the loop. Try to keep your knees together and the supporting knee (of the right leg) slightly bent. Don't arch your spine or lean forwards, sideways or backwards. Keep your abdominals pulled in, your buttocks squeezed under and your shoulders forward.

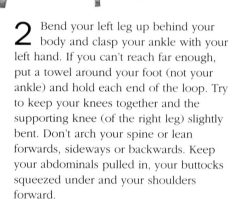

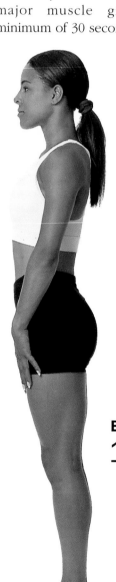

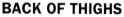

BACK OF THIGHS

1 Stand up straight with your feet close together.

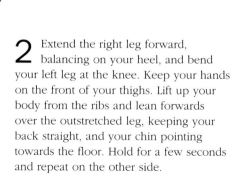

2 Extend the right leg forward, balancing on your heel, and bend your left leg at the knee. Keep your hands on the front of your thighs. Lift up your body from the ribs and lean forwards over the outstretched leg, keeping your back straight, and your chin pointing towards the floor. Hold for a few seconds and repeat on the other side.

BUTTOCKS

1 Lie on your back on the floor, with your arms by your side, palms to the floor. Bend your legs and put your feet flat on the floor.

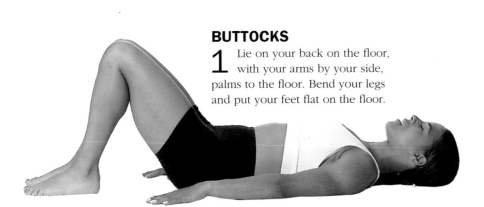

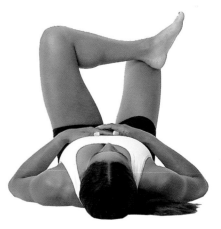

2 Rest the outside of your left foot on your right knee, letting your left knee go out at an angle to your body.

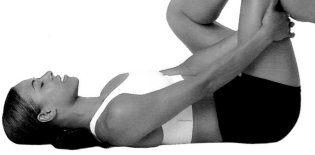

3 Grasp your right thigh with both hands and slowly lift your right foot off the floor, bringing your right knee in towards your chest. If your arms will not stretch comfortably as far as your right thigh, use a towel as a pulling loop. Change legs and repeat the exercise.

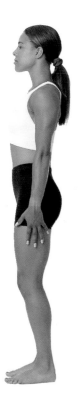

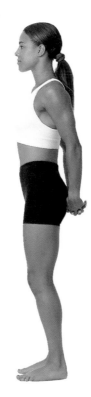

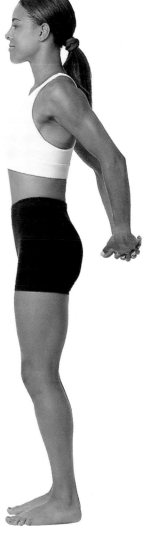

CHEST

1 Stand upright with your head raised and your feet slightly apart, in line with your shoulders.

2 Hold your arms behind you and clasp your hands together.

3 Press your shoulder blades in towards each other and slowly lift your arms up – without leaning forward. Keep your elbows slightly bent.

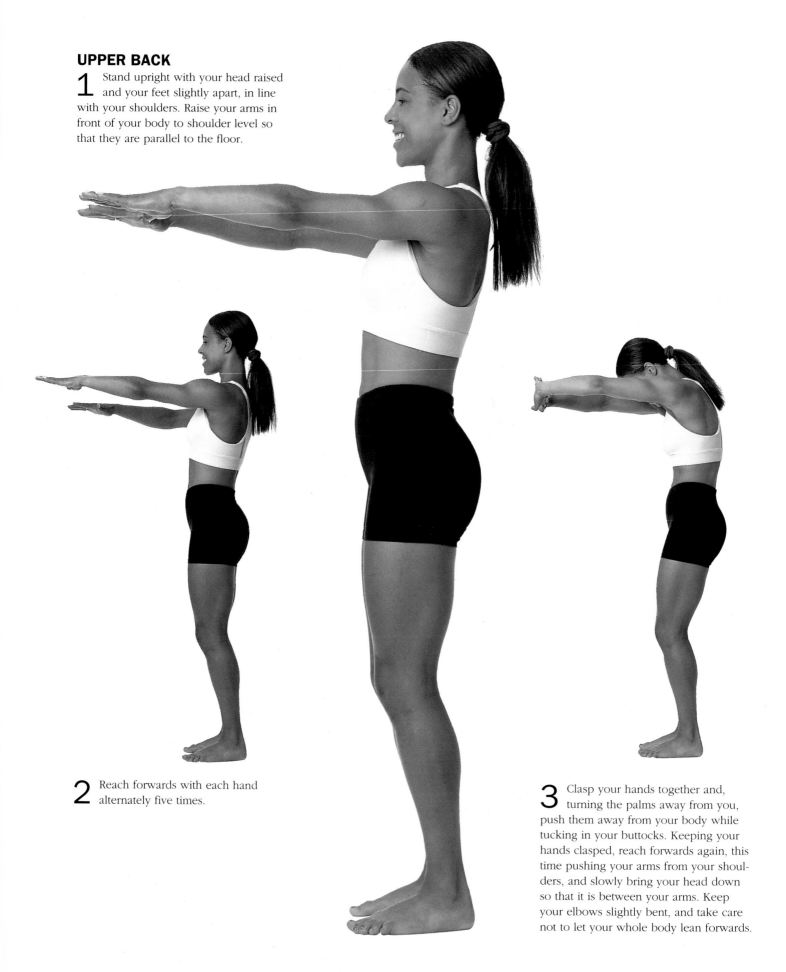

UPPER BACK

1 Stand upright with your head raised and your feet slightly apart, in line with your shoulders. Raise your arms in front of your body to shoulder level so that they are parallel to the floor.

2 Reach forwards with each hand alternately five times.

3 Clasp your hands together and, turning the palms away from you, push them away from your body while tucking in your buttocks. Keeping your hands clasped, reach forwards again, this time pushing your arms from your shoulders, and slowly bring your head down so that it is between your arms. Keep your elbows slightly bent, and take care not to let your whole body lean forwards.

LOWER BACK

This exercise is suitable for people with lower back problems as long as it is taken very gently. If you have a back problem, stop if you experience pain.

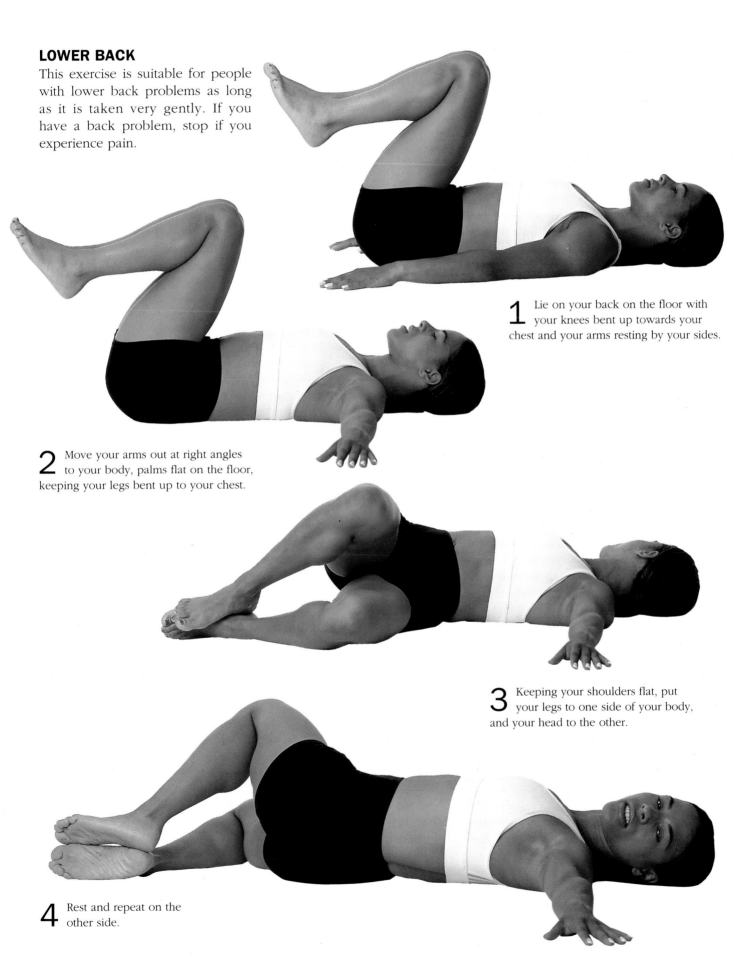

1 Lie on your back on the floor with your knees bent up towards your chest and your arms resting by your sides.

2 Move your arms out at right angles to your body, palms flat on the floor, keeping your legs bent up to your chest.

3 Keeping your shoulders flat, put your legs to one side of your body, and your head to the other.

4 Rest and repeat on the other side.

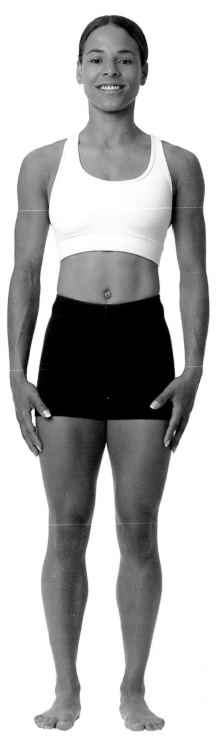

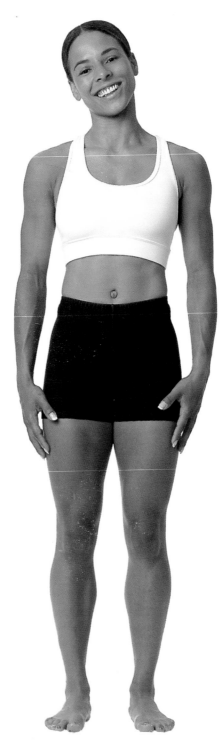

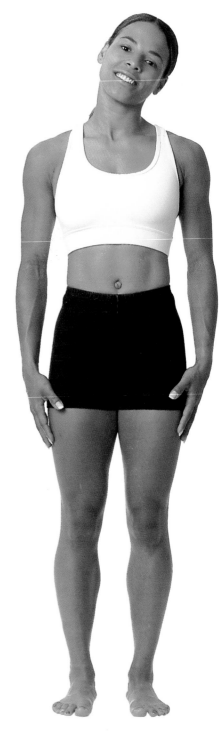

NECK AND SHOULDERS
Exercise A

1 Stand upright with your feet slightly apart, in line with your shoulders, and your shoulders back and down.

2 Ease your neck gently down to the right until you feel a slight stretch on the left side of your neck.

3 Hold, then repeat the movement to the left until you feel a gentle stretch on the right; repeat by tipping your head to the right, holding and feeling a light stretch on the left side.

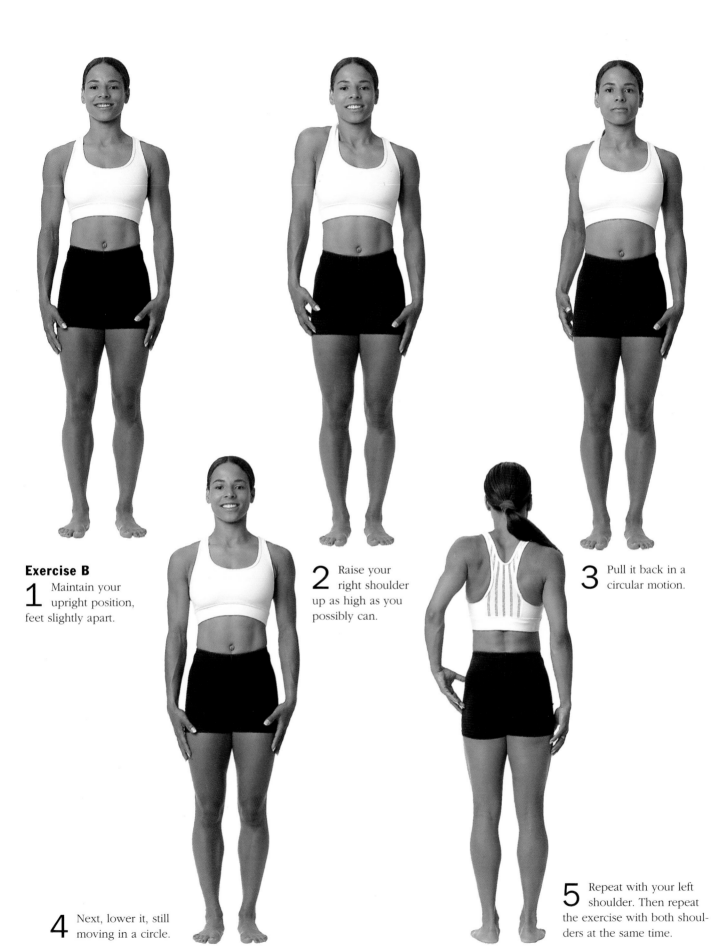

Exercise B

1 Maintain your upright position, feet slightly apart.

2 Raise your right shoulder up as high as you possibly can.

3 Pull it back in a circular motion.

4 Next, lower it, still moving in a circle.

5 Repeat with your left shoulder. Then repeat the exercise with both shoulders at the same time.

HEALTHY EATING AND DIETING

A WELL-BALANCED DIET IS THE SECRET TO BEING IN GOOD HEALTH AND GREAT SHAPE. BUT EATING WELL DOES NOT MEAN YOU HAVE TO BUY PRICEY OUT-OF-SEASON FOOD OR COOK TIME-CONSUMING MEALS. IF YOUR CURRENT DIET IS LOPSIDED, BE PRACTICAL ABOUT REVAMPING IT: TASTEBUDS THAT ARE ACCUSTOMED TO FAST AND FRIED FOODS ARE NOT GOING TO BE STIMULATED BY FRESH FRUIT AND FIBRE OVERNIGHT. THE SAME GOES FOR WEIGHT-LOSS DIETS: BE REALISTIC ABOUT YOUR AIMS AND DO NOT BE TOO TOUGH ON YOURSELF — IT IS NOT A CRIME TO ENJOY FORBIDDEN FOODS FROM TIME TO TIME. YOU WILL HAVE NO PROBLEM LOSING WEIGHT QUICKLY IF YOU COMBINE REGULAR EXERCISE WITH A LOW FAT DIET BASED ON THE TASTY, EASY-TO-PREPARE RECIPES INCLUDED IN THIS SECTION.

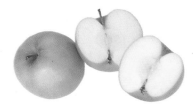

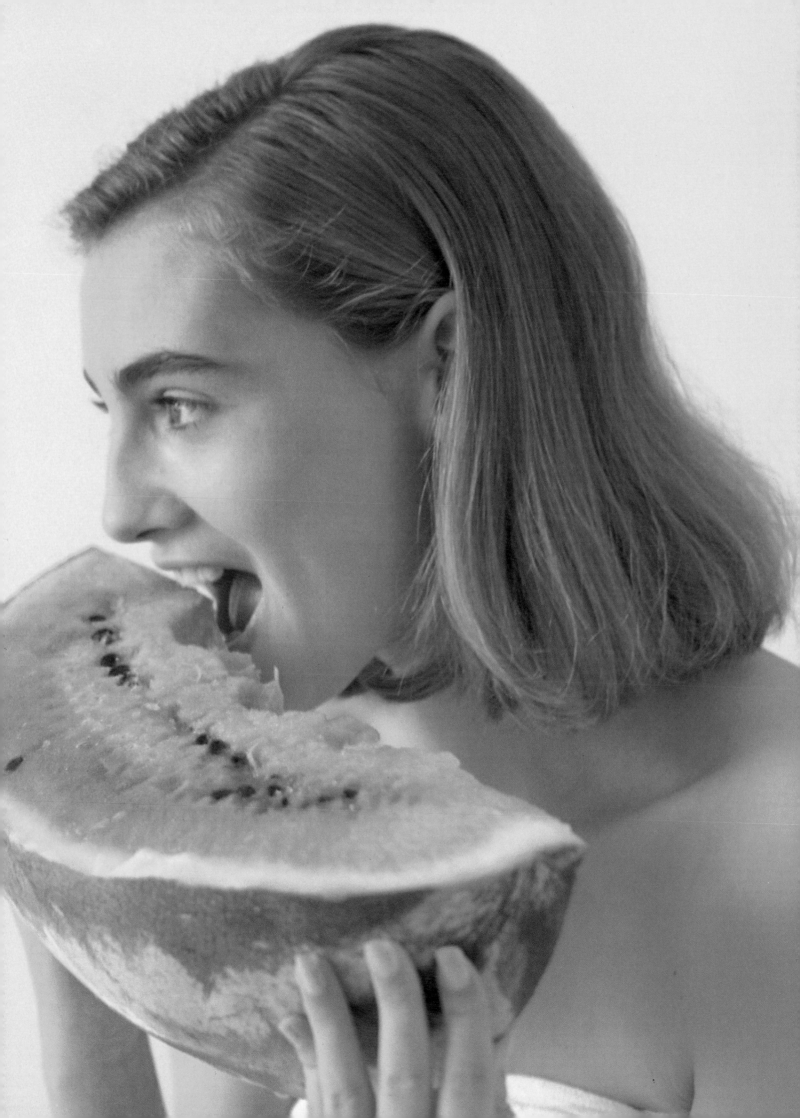

DIET FOR LIFE

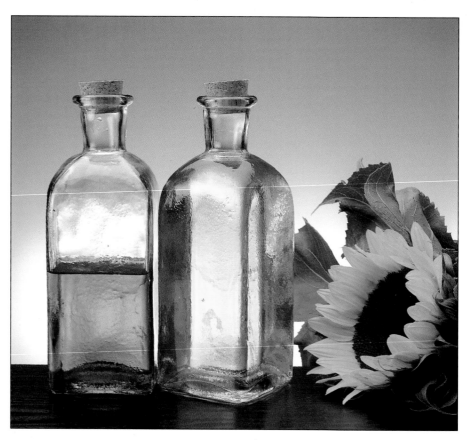

Eat monounsaturated fats such as olive oil, and polyunsaturates such as sunflower oil, in preference to butter and other saturated fats.

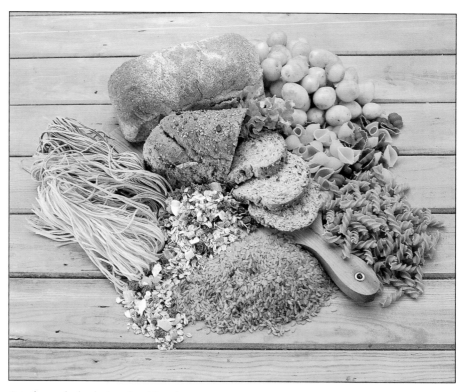

Starchy carbohydrates should make up about 50 per cent of the daily diet.

Balance is important to a healthy diet. The way we eat affects our well-being, so knowing how to choose a healthy combination of foods is the first step towards improving our eating habits and lifestyle.

FAT – FRIEND AND FOE

Eggs, butter, milk, and meat are a good source of energy, but we tend to eat too much fat which is why many of us are overweight: fat produces fat. Cut down on fat in your diet but do not cut it out completely: eat less fatty red meat and more fish and poultry; grill, bake, or stir-fry (using polyunsaturated and monounsaturated oils), eat eggs in moderation, and use semi-skimmed or skimmed milk instead of full-fat milk. Try to use margarine, or try switching to a reduced fat olive-oil spread instead of butter; if you like butter, reserve it for special occasions.

Saturated fats come mainly from animal products (milk, butter, cheese, and meat) and in excess are thought to contribute to raised cholesterol levels.

Polyunsaturated fats are found in vegetable oils such as sunflower, safflower, corn, and soya bean oils; they are also found in some fish oils and some nuts, and are said to help lower cholesterol levels.

Monounsaturated fats are found in olive and rapeseed oils; they are also said to lower cholesterol levels.

GRAINS, FRUIT, AND VEGETABLES

Eat plenty of wholegrain foods such as brown rice, wholemeal bread, wholemeal flour, and wholemeal pasta; they should form the bulk of a healthy diet. Also concentrate on eating lots of fresh fruit and vegetables: these are rich in carbohydrates, minerals, and vitamins. To obtain all of these nutrients, try to eat as many raw vegetables as possible.

SUGAR SWEET

Many of us tend to eat too much sugar so try cutting added sugar out of your diet completely for 21 days (your body will still obtain it naturally from certain vegetables and fruit) and see how you feel: even if you are not actively dieting you will probably find that you lose some weight. Craving sugary foods such as doughnuts and pastries when you are pre-menstrual is common in some women. One way of combating this is to eat little and often; snack on fruit with a high water content, such as watermelon and strawberries.

SALTY ISSUES

Even if you are not dieting you should eat less salt as it may lead to high blood pressure. There are some good low-sodium salts available, so use these instead of the real thing if you do need to season food with salt. Do not buy salted butter, avoid processed and smoked cheeses, add the barest minimum of salt (or none at all) to cooking water, and avoid processed foods.

FLUID INTAKE

Drink plenty of water: your body loses between 2-3 litres/3-5 pints of fluid every day, so drink no less than 1.5 litres/2½ pints of water daily. Once you get into the swing of it, consciously drinking water is an easy habit to maintain. Just keep some to hand and sip it slowly throughout the day.

HEALTHY DIET CHECKLIST

The healthy eating guidelines summarized here are not difficult to apply to a daily diet. Once you

FIBRE FACTS

Fibre is important to a healthy diet. Your body cannot digest it, so, in rather basic terms, it goes in and comes out, taking other waste with it. Fibrous foods include bread, rice, cereals, vegetables, fruit, and nuts. We should aim for about 30 g (just over 1 oz) of fibre a day. These are some examples of good fibre sources:

Good Sources	Average Portion	Grams of Fibre
wholemeal pasta	75 g/3 oz (uncooked)	9
baked beans	125 g/4 oz	8
frozen peas	75 g/3 oz	8
bran flakes	50 g/2 oz	7
muesli	50 g/2 oz	4-5
raspberries	100 g/3½ oz	6
blackberries	100 g/3½ oz	6
banana	average fruit	3.5
baked jacket potato	150 g/ 5 oz	3.5
brown rice	50 g/2 oz	3
cabbage	100 g/3½ oz	3
red kidney beans	40 g/1½ oz	3
wholemeal bread	1 large slice	3
high-fibre white bread	1 large slice	2
stewed prunes	6 fruit	2

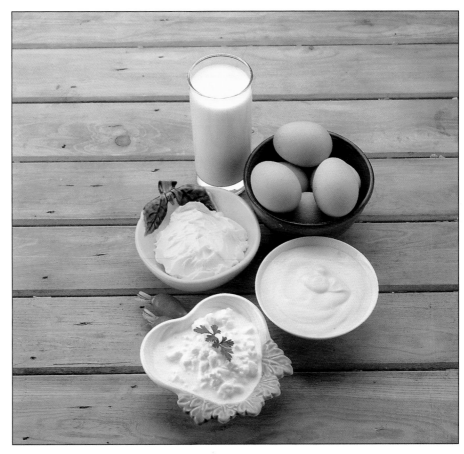

Dairy products such as egg yolks, hard cheeses, and full fat milk contain high levels of fat. Choose low fat milks, cheeses, and yogurts.

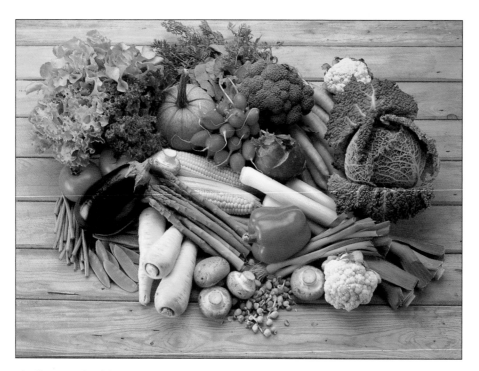

Ideally, you should eat at least two portions of vegetables – fresh, frozen, or tinned – with your main meal.

have adopted them, they will become part of your daily routine so there is no reason why you cannot follow a healthy diet for the rest of your life.

❍ Eat lots of fresh fruit and vegetables, ideally five portions, or about 398 g/14 oz a day.

❍ Be wary of the amount of fat you eat.

❍ Try to eat half your daily food in the form of starchy carbohydrates such as potatoes, bread, pasta and rice.

❍ Replace refined flour with wholemeal flour.

❍ Eat more fibre-rich foods such as wholemeal bread and pasta, brown rice and pulses.

❍ Cut down on sugar.

❍ Cut down on salt.

❍ Drink lots of water; reduce coffee and tea. The caffeine they

VITAMIN VALUES

Vitamin	Sources include	Benefits
Vitamin A	liver (especially fish livers), egg yolk, fortified margarine, oily fish, oranges, apricots, carrots, tomatoes, melons, dark green leafy vegetables	eye sight; skin; may protect against cancer
Vitamin B_1	most foods – including wheatgerm and pulses, whole grains, brewer's yeast, nuts, fortified breakfast cereals	helps break down carbohydrates; nervous system
Vitamin B_2	brewer's yeast, liver, kidney, dairy produce, wheat bran, wheatgerm, eggs	repairs body tissues
Vitamin B_3	wheatgerm, whole grain cereals, meat, fish	essential for tissue chemical reactions
Vitamin B_6	avocados, liver, whole grains, egg yolk, lean meat, bananas, fish, potatoes	nervous system; skin; red blood cells
Vitamin B_{12}	liver, kidney, some fish (including shellfish), eggs, milk	healthy blood and nerves
Vitamin C	citrus fruits, potatoes, tomatoes, leafy greens	helps heal wounds, may fight colds, 'flu and infections; protects gums, keeps joints and ligaments in good working order
Vitamin D	fish liver oils, fatty fish, eggs, fortified margarine also synthesized by ultraviolet light	calcium deposits in bones
Vitamin E	vegetable oils, some vegetables, wheatgerm	cell growth; antioxidant
Vitamin K	most vegetables – especially leafy greens ones, liver	essential in production of some proteins

contain is stimulating, so try swapping them for herbal teas. If you cannot give up coffee switch to organic Arabica beans, which can be brewed instead of instant granular coffee – and limit yourself to two cups a day.

○ Cut down on sugary canned drinks and particularly on alcohol intake. It is very important to cut down on alcohol if you drink more than 14 units a week (for a woman); 14 units is equivalent to 2 glasses of wine a day.

IDEAL WEEKLY FOOD QUOTA

Eat food from each of the four main food groups each day.

○ Starchy foods, including bread, cereals, pasta, potatoes and rice.

○ Dairy products (preferably low fat).

○ Meat, fish, poultry, beans and lentils, nuts, and eggs.

○ Vegetables and fruit.

Some authorities, such as the World Health Organization, recommend eating 5 portions a day from this group; this is thought to help prevent cancer.

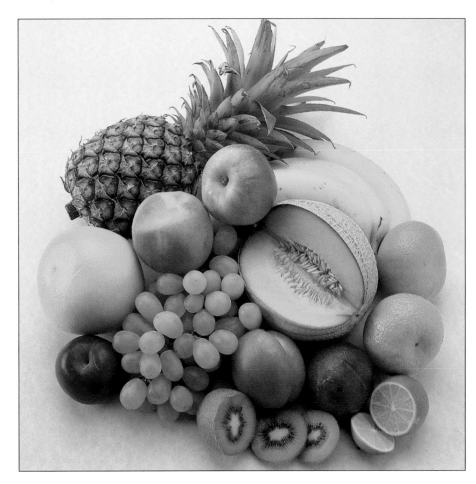

Fresh fruit makes a healthy, low calorie snack food that is filling as well as delicious.

VALUABLE MINERALS

As well as vitamins, a wide variety of minerals are essential for good health, growth, and body functioning. Some, such as calcium and iron, are needed in quite large amounts, and for some people there is a real risk of deficiency if they do not eat a healthy diet.

Calcium: A regular supply of calcium is vital because bone tissue is constantly being broken down and rebuilt. A calcium-rich diet is particularly important during adolescence, pregnancy, breast-feeding, the menopause, and for the elderly. Smoking, lack of exercise, too much alcohol, high protein and high salt intakes all encourage calcium losses.

Iron: Only a fraction of the iron present in food is absorbed, although it is much more readily absorbed from red meat than from vegetable sources. Vitamin C also helps with absorption. Pregnant women, women who have heavy periods, and vegetarians should all be particularly careful about ensuring an adequate intake.

Trace elements: These include other essential minerals such as zinc, iodine, magnesium, and potassium. Although important, they are only needed in minute quantities. They are found in a wide variety of foods and deficiency is very rare.

Mineral	Sources	Essential for
Calcium	cheese, milk, yogurt, eggs, bread, nuts, pulses, fish with soft bones such as whitebait and tinned sardines, leafy green vegetables	healthy bones, teeth and nails; muscle and nerve function; blood clotting; milk production in nursing mothers
Iron	liver, red meat, oily fish, whole grain cereals, leafy green vegetables	makes haemoglobin, the pigment in red bloods cells that helps transport oxygen around the body

EATING FOR ENERGY

How often do you feel tired and lethargic? Does your energy dip dramatically in the afternoons making you feel dozy (even if you have not washed down a three-course lunch with a bottle of wine) and in need of 40 winks? If you life is regularly disrupted by fatigue and you want to take action, one of the wisest things to do is to look at your diet and, if necessary, change what you eat and how you eat it.

OFF TO A GOOD START
There is logic behind the saying "breakfast like a king, lunch like a prince and dine like a pauper." If you start the day with a substantial breakfast your body will be getting all the energy it needs early on.

CHANGING YOUR EATING HABITS
You are most likely to succeed in changing your diet if you eat regularly, in moderation, and slowly – and savour every mouthful. Although the bonuses of eating in a balanced way do not come instantly, if you take stock now and concentrate on eating the fresh foods suggested below, as well as avoiding high-fat, sugar-rich foods such as cakes, pastries, and salty snacks, you will probably notice a marked difference in your energy levels within a couple of weeks.

VITALITY FOODS FOR EXTRA ENERGY
A diet that makes you feel more energetic is based on natural, wholesome foods that are nutritious, rather than fatty and fast foods. If you want to boost your energy levels, stock up on fresh and dried fruits that are high in natural sugars such as pears, kiwi fruit, and apricots, vegetables such as peas, spinach, cabbage, and

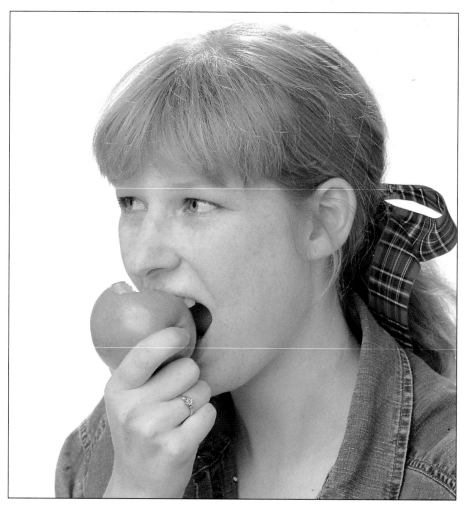

onions, and oily fish, poultry, and red meats such as game and lean beef. Eat nuts, brown rice, seeds, pulses, wheatgerm, whole-grains, and foods that contain minerals such as magnesium, phosphorus, and zinc, and water-soluble vitamins B and C. Use cold-pressed oils such as grapeseed, olive, sesame, sunflower, hazelnut, and walnut to dress salads; do not skip dairy foods but use milk and natural yogurt (preferably low fat); replace sliced white loaves with bread made from wholemeal flour.

SUPER SQUEEZES AND SHAKES
Home-made fruit juices and milk- or yogurt-based drinks are energy-boosting alternatives to commercially prepared drinks, and are easy

Nutritionists and other health professionals recommend eating fresh fruit every day.

to prepare. Choose sweet fruits such as mango, banana, and apricots – these have a naturally high sugar content – switch on the juicer or liquidizer and drink them chilled. Here are two sparkling shakes to try:

1 mango
2 slices pineapple
1 banana
150 ml/5 fl oz semi-skimmed or skimmed milk or a small carton of natural low fat yogurt
2.5 ml/¹/₂ tsp honey (optional)
or:
a handful of raspberries and strawberries
2 apricots
100 ml/4 fl oz milk or natural low fat yogurt

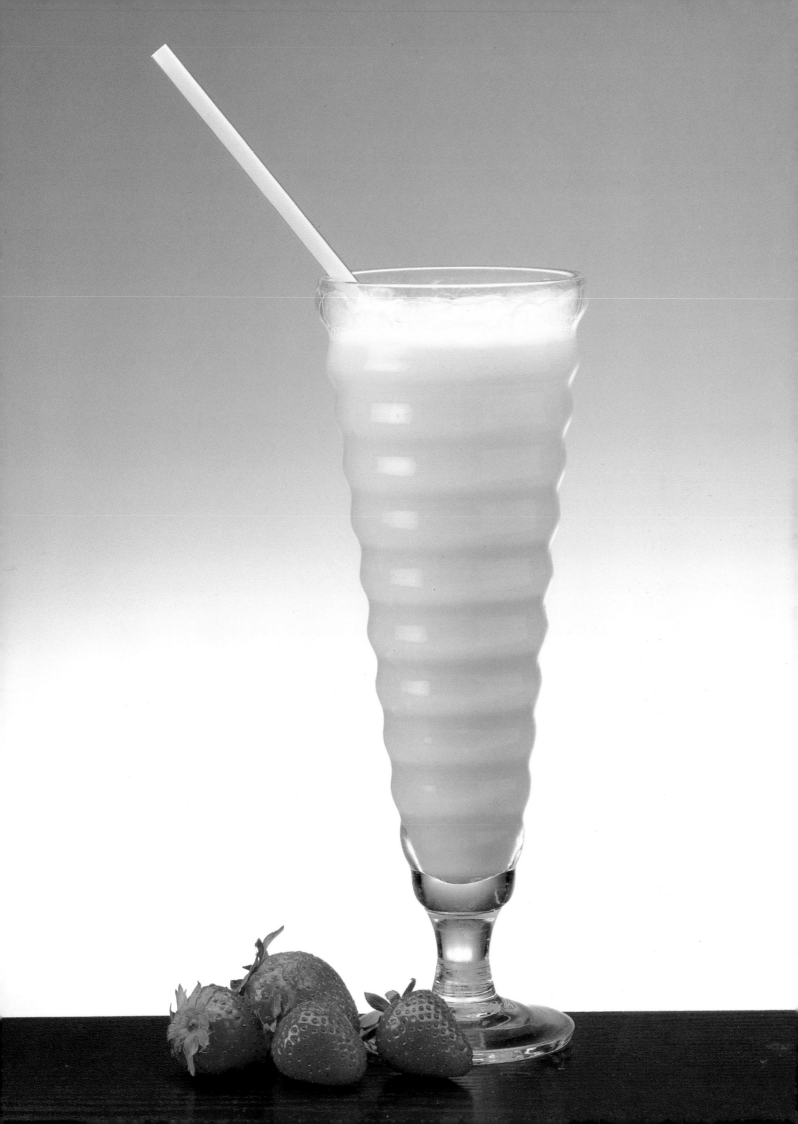

DIET AND WEIGHT LOSS

People tackle weight loss in ways that suit their lifestyles. But the safest and best way to shift excess pounds is to combine regular exercise with a balanced calorie-controlled diet. What you eat when you are trying to take off weight should not be that different from a normal eating plan – except for the amount you consume. If you only have a small amount to lose and you cut your calorie intake by 1000 from the recommended 2300 calories per day, you will lose weight; if you are aiming to lose a significant amount, stick to 1200 calories a day and you will get there. Your basic weight loss ethos is less sugar and saturated fats, more fibre and starch; the calories you eat should come from foods that supply you with the right number of nutrients to keep your body functioning properly.

MIND OVER MATTER

Quick weight loss is inspiring, but it is important to think ahead too: you need to retrain your palate and eating habits and reassess your physical activity so that you can lose weight and stay slim. You cannot expect to achieve miracles in a few days, but you will see a difference within three or four weeks if you eat properly and exercise regularly. Losing weight successfully is like getting fitter: you need a horizon – or goal – ahead of you to help spur you on.

ABSOLUTELY AVOID

Chocolate, biscuits, doughnuts, fizzy drinks, cakes, ice cream, sugared cereals – in fact anything that contains refined sugar, it's just empty calories: a confectionary bar, for instance, has 230 calories and has absolutely no food value.

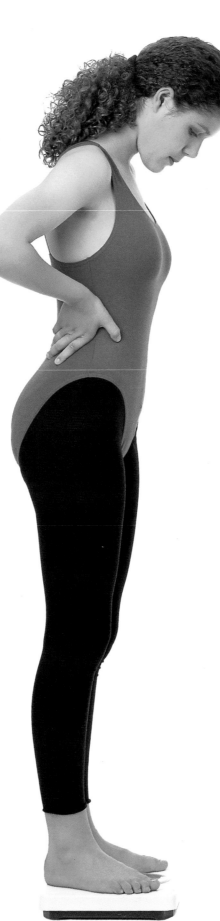

SLIMMERS' TIPS

○ If you can, eat more at the start of the day to give you energy and time to burn off the calories.
○ Eat little and often to stop hunger pangs.
○ Drink lots of water.
○ If you want to snack, keep a supply of raw fruit, vegetables, and raisins nearby.
○ Don't be tempted to take slimming pills, diuretics, or laxatives to speed up weight loss; they upset the body's natural equilibrium – something that can take considerable time to rebalance.
○ Exercise regularly; extra activity uses up calories, and this is essential to weight loss.
○ Don't give up if you lapse: it is quite normal to veer off track every so often, and as long as you get back on course as soon as you can, all your hard work will not be ruined.

HOW MUCH WEIGHT CAN I LOSE?

To lose weight you have to eat fewer calories than your body burns up every day, but the amount varies from person to person. The exact amount depends on your personal composition – how much fat your body has, your metabolism, and the amount you weigh to begin with. As a rule of thumb though, the heavier you are when you start slimming, the more weight you are likely to lose within 21 days or a month. When you lose weight it comes off all areas of your body, but it can take longer to shift from certain areas, such as your arms and legs. This is where exercise is particularly helpful: working on specific trouble spots will encourage the weight to come off more quickly.

Left: Don't be tempted to weigh yourself too often – once every 10 days is enough.

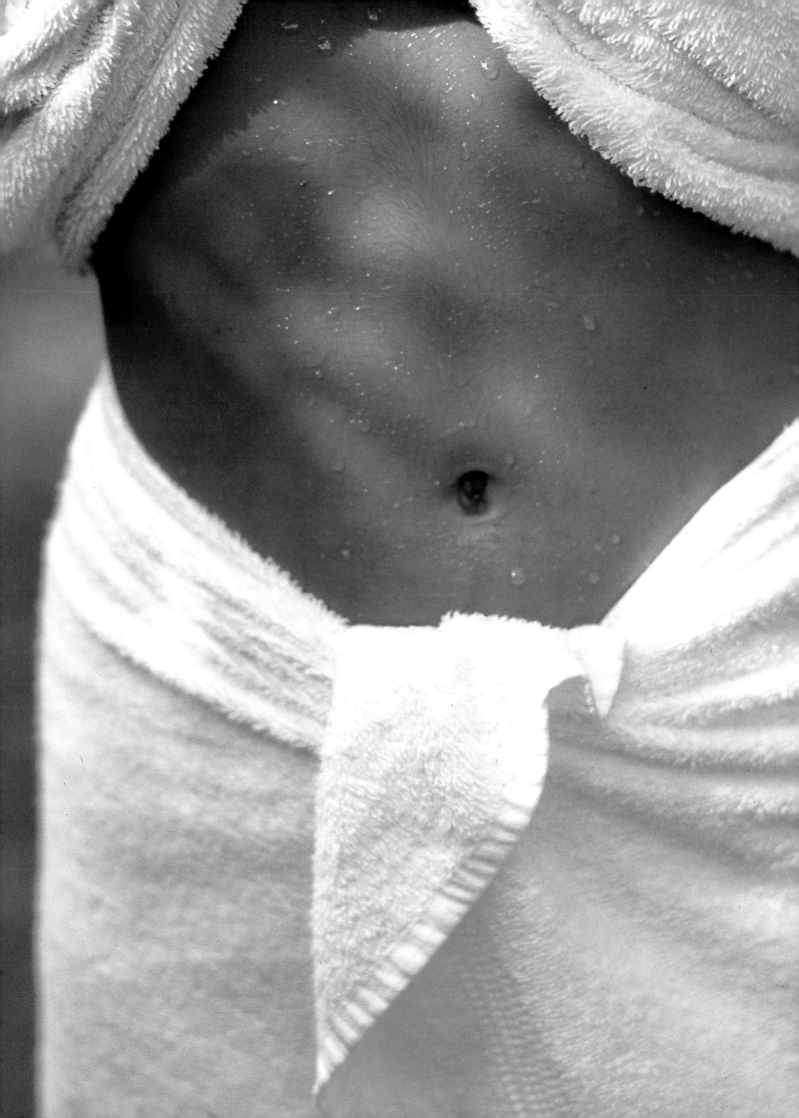

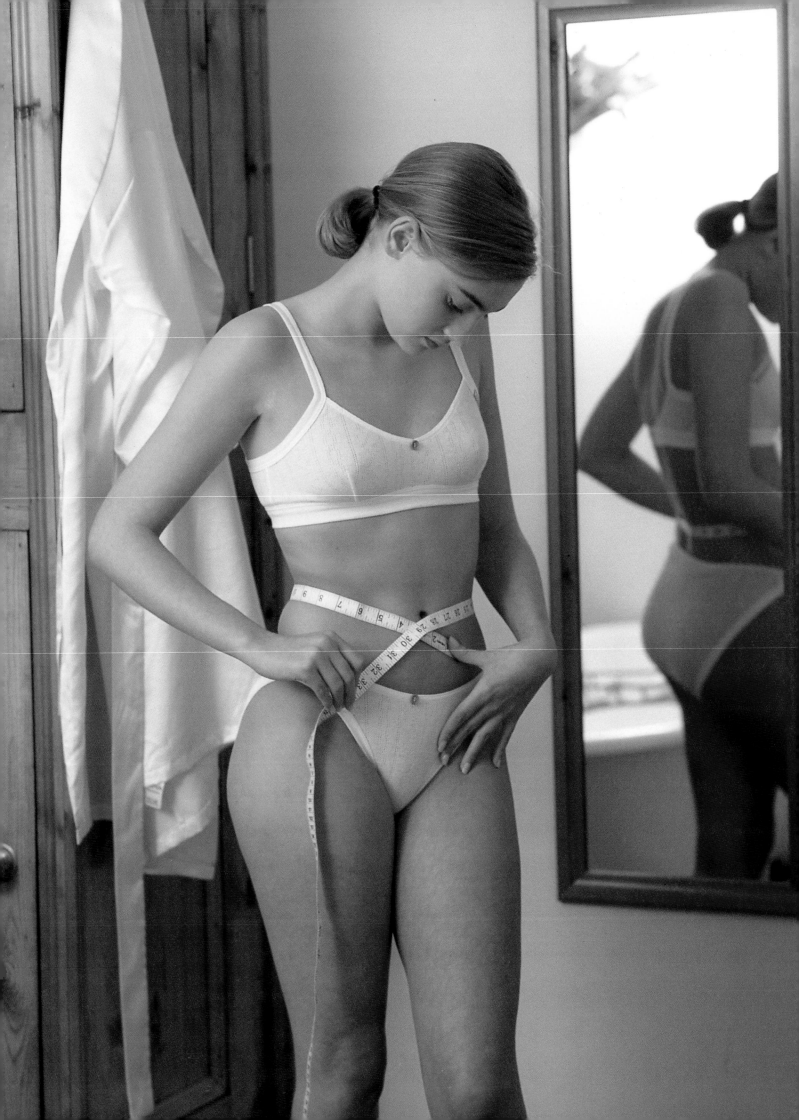

MYTH-BREAKER:
If I Stop Smoking Will I Gain Weight?

You may well put on a small amount of weight at first but if you are serious about getting fitter you have absolutely no choice but to kick smoking. Tobacco is toxic. If you are a smoker, stopping is the biggest leap you can make towards living a healthier lifestyle; if you are following a straightforward weight-loss diet and think that kicking the habit will make you pick at food all day, keep lots of raw vegetables and raisins on hand to munch on.

EATING OUT – AND STAYING ON COURSE

The problem of what to do when dieting and eating out is a tricky one. At the height of the 1980s' slimming boom, some restaurants offered specific diet options on their menus, but few give this kind of service now that dieting is less fashionable. The best way to get around the problem of dining out without lapsing – without drawing attention to yourself and still being able to enjoy yourself – is as follows:

❍ Order a salad starter.

❍ Skip bread or breadsticks, or eat a piece of bread without butter - it can be just as delicious.

MYTH-BREAKER:
If I Skip Meals Will I Lose Weight More Quickly?

Do not be tempted to skip meals. Skipping meals makes you crave, overeat at the next meal, and it slows down your metabolism, which ultimately hinders weight loss.

Left: Keeping an accurate record of your measurements is one way of calculating weight loss.

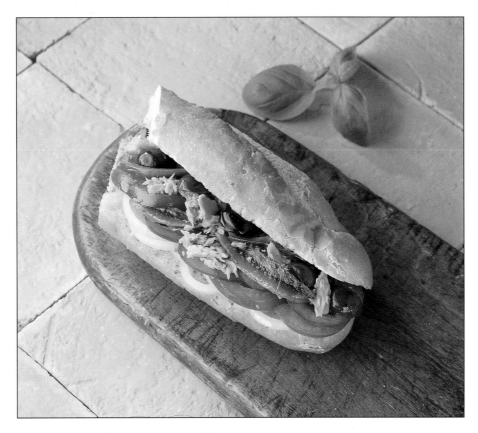

❍ Drink one glass of wine, and lots of water.

❍ Choose a simple main course, something like grilled fish or chicken; avoid anything that is drenched in a rich sauce or in lots of butter.

❍ Choose a simple low fat dessert: a sorbet is ideal.

❍ Finish with herbal tea (peppermint is very refreshing and settles your stomach after eating); or, if you have to have a coffee, choose espresso or black coffee, not cappuccino.

GAUGING WEIGHT LOSS

You may choose to weigh yourself once a week first thing in the morning. Drawing up a goal chart to record any weight losses (and gains) may help to keep you inspired. Or, if you prefer, ignore the scales and just focus on how you feel by keeping a check on how your clothes feel. When tight clothes become more comfortable

A sandwich with fresh ingredients makes a healthy lunch – even for weight watchers.

this is a sure sign that you are losing weight. Alternatively, you may prefer to keep a record of your measurements (bust, waist, and hips) and see how they alter over the 21-day period. Do whatever works for you, and when you have lost a little weight reward yourself with a special calorie-free treat such as a new lipstick, eyeshadow, or a manicure.

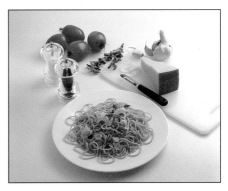

Nutritious, starchy foods such as pasta are not fattening if eaten with low fat sauces.

RECIPES FOR HEALTHY EATING

Whether you are slimming or just trying to change your eating habits for the better, the key to a healthy diet is variety – not just in terms of taste but also in the range of foods you eat. Diets that are based on one or two types of food – for example fruit or vegetables – impose a rigid routine that quickly becomes boring and will probably result in your lapsing; more important, such diets are also unhealthy. The recipes on the following pages are based on the foods needed to maintain good health, and have also been developed for those wishing to lose weight by following a calorie-controlled diet. Nutritional information specific to each dish is given with each recipe, together with a calorie count per portion, so that you know exactly what you are getting out of your food.

DIETER'S GUIDELINES

Given the modern, more sedentary lifestyle of the majority of people, the recommended calorie intake for men and women who are not over-weight is around 2300 calories a day. If you are overweight and want to lose weight fairly quickly you should cut down by 1100 calories, making your daily intake 1200 calories. If you want to lose weight more slowly, you can allow yourself a daily intake of 1500 calories. If you exercise regularly as well as keeping calories within these ranges, it is possible to lose around 0.7 kg/1 1/2 lb a week.

EAT WELL AND LOSE WEIGHT

An intake of 1200 or 1500 calories a day does not mean that you have to limit yourself to just a few foods as the following examples demonstrate. The two examples of daily menus given below show you just how appetizing, satisfying, and varied your calorie-controlled diet can be.

IMPORTANT NOTE
The number of calories given for the suggested menus can only be approximate because the actual number depends on the weight of each portion. If you are following a calorie-controlled diet it is essential that you make use of a calorie counter and accurate kitchen scales.

Those dishes marked with an asterisk (*) are included in the recipe section beginning on the next page.

MENU ONE: 1200 CALORIES
For this and the next menu you can drink as much as you like of these beverages: black tea and coffee, herbal tea, hot water with a squeeze of lemon juice, and water.

Breakfast
25 g/1 oz muesli with 15 ml/1 tbsp low fat natural yogurt
1 banana

Mid-morning
Tea or coffee with 30 ml/2 tbsp milk

Lunch
*Red Coleslaw**
1 baked potato with 1 portion of low fat natural cottage cheese

Mid-afternoon
Black tea or coffee
*Applenut Cookie**

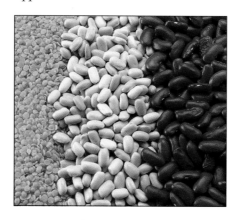

Dinner
*Pork Steaks with Peppercorn Glaze**
portion of steamed brown rice
*Baked Spiced Plums with Ricotta**

MENU TWO: 1500 CALORIES
Many people are in the habit of eating a light lunch and big dinner, but if it is convenient you could have a large lunch and light dinner, as in this suggested daily menu: the important thing is to make sure you don't take in more than the recommended number of calories for the day.

Breakfast
1/2 grapefruit
1 serving bran flakes with semi-skimmed milk
1 thick slice wholemeal toast with low fat spread
small spoonful of reduced-sugar jam or marmalade
tea or coffee with milk

Mid-morning
tea or coffee with milk
1 apple

Lunch
*Spicy Chicken Provençale**
one portion steamed broccoli
one portion new potatoes
1 low fat fruit yogurt

Mid-afternoon
*1 slice of Spiced Carrot and Sultana Loaf**
glass of semi-skimmed milk

Dinner
*Golden Pepper and Orange Soup**
*Spinach, Apricot, and Hazelnut Salad**
*Savoury Bread Knot**

Pulses are very nutritious, have a high fibre content, and are an excellent source of low fat protein for those preferring a vegetarian diet.

STARTERS

TUNA, DILL, AND LIME DIP

A light, refreshing dip to serve with crisp vegetable crudités.

Serves: 4   *Preparation time:* 5 minutes

200 g/7 oz can tuna fish in brine, drained
45 ml/3 tbsp Greek-style yogurt
finely grated rind 1/2 lime
15 ml/1 tbsp chopped fresh dill
salt and black pepper

1 Place the tuna fish and yogurt in a blender and process for a few seconds until almost smooth. Alternatively, mash thoroughly with a fork.

2 Stir in the lime rind, dill, and seasoning to taste.

3 Spoon into a small dish and serve with sticks of raw vegetables for dipping.

All calorie values are for the recipes only and do not include any serving suggestions.

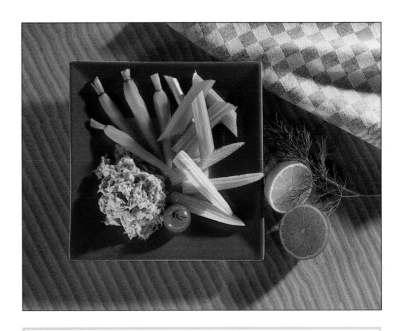

70 CALORIES A PORTION

Using drained tuna in brine, rather than tuna in oil, makes this a low fat recipe. Raw vegetable crudités, particularly carrots for Vitamin A (as beta-carotene) and raw pepper, celery, courgette, or cauliflower florets for Vitamin C, will provide a good vitamin contribution.

SWEETCORN AND CHIVE RAMEKINS

These little soufflés are light as air and very simple to make.

Serves: 6   *Preparation time:* 5 minutes
Cooking time: 8–10 minutes

3 eggs, separated
200 g/7 oz can sweetcorn, drained
45 ml/3 tbsp snipped fresh chives
45 ml/3 tbsp fresh wholemeal breadcrumbs
15 ml/1 tbsp grated Parmesan cheese
salt and black pepper

1 Preheat the oven to 200°C/400°F/Gas 6. Stir together the egg yolks, sweetcorn, chives, and breadcrumbs. Season well.

2 Whisk the egg whites until stiff, then fold them evenly into the corn mixture. Spoon into six small ramekin dishes.

3 Sprinkle with Parmesan cheese, place on a baking sheet and bake for 8–10 minutes until well-risen and golden brown. Serve immediately.

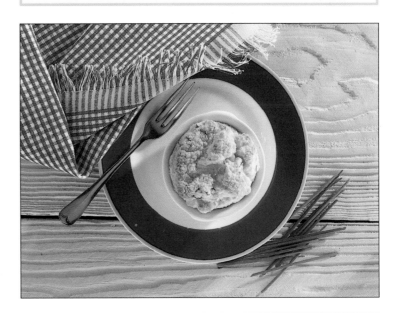

80 CALORIES A PORTION

This recipe provides valuable amounts of fibre, both from the sweetcorn and the wholemeal breadcrumbs. Hard cheeses, such as Parmesan, are high in fat, but because this is a strong-tasting cheese you only need use a little for a lot of flavour. Eggs too are very nourishing, providing vitamins A, B, and D, iron and protein.

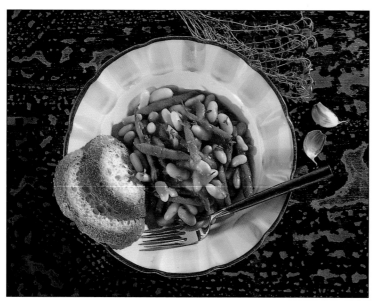

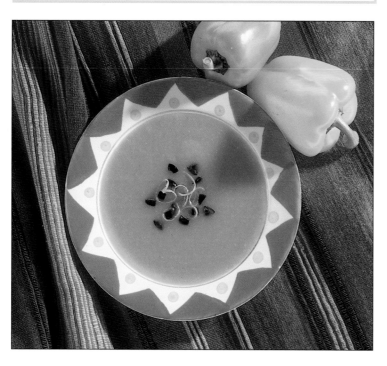

MIXED BEANS IN PASSATA

An easy but filling snack or starter. Vary the beans to include your favourites.

Serves: 4   *Preparation time:* 5 minutes
Cooking time: 15–18 minutes

5 ml/1 tsp olive oil
1 medium red onion, finely chopped
2 garlic cloves, crushed
150 ml/^{1}/$_4$ pint/^{2}/$_3$ cup passata
2 large sprigs fresh or dried thyme
115 g/4 oz/1^1/$_2$ cups frozen or fresh French beans
432 g/15 oz can cannelini beans
salt and black pepper

1 Heat the olive oil and fry the onion and garlic gently for 10 minutes until softened but not browned.

2 Add the passata and thyme and bring to the boil. Add the French beans, then cover and simmer gently for 5–8 minutes until tender.

3 Add the cannelini beans, season well and serve with thin slices of wholemeal toast.

GOLDEN PEPPER AND ORANGE SOUP

This virtually fat free, golden soup makes a surprisingly light starter.

Serves: 4   *Preparation time:* 15 minutes
Cooking time: about 15 minutes

3 yellow or orange (bell) peppers, halved and seeded
1 large onion, chopped
grated rind and juice of 1 large orange
350 ml/12 fl oz/1^1/$_2$ cups chicken stock
4 stoned black olives, chopped
salt and black pepper

1 Place the peppers, skin side up, on a baking sheet. Cook under a hot grill until the skins are blackened. Cover and leave to cool.

2 Place the onion in a pan with the orange juice. Bring to the boil, then cover and simmer gently for 10 minutes or until the onion is tender.

3 Peel the peppers. Purée in a blender with onion, half the orange rind, and chicken stock until smooth.

4 Season well, then heat gently. Serve sprinkled with olives and the remaining orange rind.

CHICKEN AND MUSHROOM TERRINE

A light, low-fat starter.

Serves: 4   *Preparation time:* 15 minutes
Cooking time: 45–50 minutes

2 shallots, chopped
175 g/6 oz/2 cups mush-
   rooms, chopped
45 ml/3 tbsp chicken stock
2 chicken breasts without
   skin, chopped
1 egg white
30 ml/2 tbsp wholemeal
   breadcrumbs
salt and black pepper
30 ml/2 tbsp chopped
   fresh parsley
30 ml/2 tbsp chopped
   sage

1 Preheat the oven to 180°C/350°F/Gas 4. Place the shallots, mushrooms, and chicken stock in a pan and cook gently, stirring occasionally, until the vegetables have softened and the mixture is dry.

2 Place in a food processor with the chicken breasts, egg white, breadcrumbs, and seasoning and chop coarsely. Add the chopped herbs. Spoon into a greased 900 ml/1$\frac{1}{2}$ pint/3$\frac{3}{4}$ cup loaf tin and smooth the surface.

3 Cover with foil and bake for 35–40 minutes, until the juices are no longer pink. Place a weight on top, leave to cool, then chill. Serve sliced.

ROAST TOMATO AND CHICKPEA SOUP

This unusual soup is cooked in the oven for a rich, roasted flavour.

Serves: 4   *Preparation time:* 10 minutes
Cooking time: 30 minutes

6 large plum tomatoes
1 medium onion, halved
2 garlic cloves
300 ml/$\frac{1}{2}$ pint/1$\frac{1}{4}$ cups vegetable stock
430 g can chickpeas, drained
30 ml/2 tbsp tomato purée
30 ml/2 tbsp chopped fresh coriander
salt and black pepper

1 Preheat the oven to 200°C/400°F/Gas 6. Place the whole tomatoes, onion, and garlic on a baking sheet and bake for 30 minutes until tender and lightly browned.

2 Place in a food processor with the vegetable stock and half the chickpeas, and blend until smooth. Press through a sieve.

3 Return to the pan, add the tomato purée, the remaining chickpeas, and the coriander. Bring to the boil and serve hot.

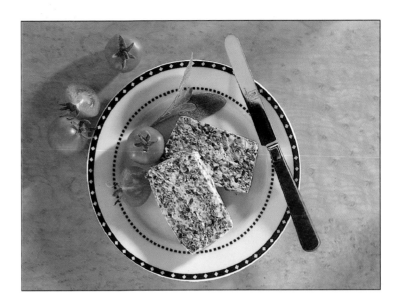

95 CALORIES A PORTION

Cooking mushrooms in stock is an excellent way of incorporating the delicious mushroom flavour into a recipe without dramatically increasing the fat content, as would happen if cooked in butter. Mushrooms provide B vitamins and some fibre. Always skin poultry prior to cooking to maintain a low fat content.

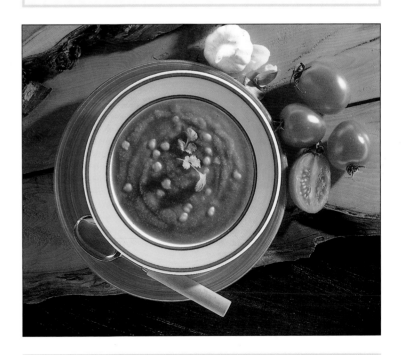

80 CALORIES A PORTION

Tomatoes are an excellent source of Vitamin C but do not over-heat this soup or keep it warm, since Vitamin C is rapidly destroyed on heating. The chickpeas also add plenty of fibre.

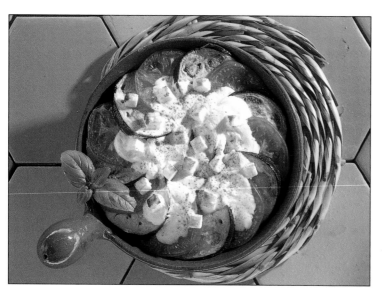

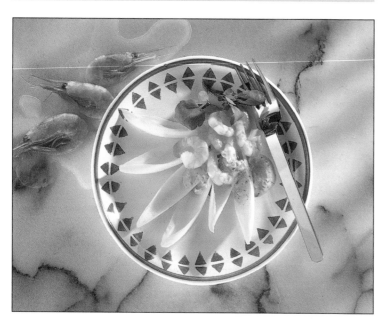

BAKED AUBERGINES, TOMATOES AND FETA

Aubergines usually absorb lots of oil during cooking, but when cooked this way they are relatively low in fat.

Serves: 4   *Preparation time:* 5 minutes, plus 30 minutes standing time   *Cooking time:* 25–30 minutes

1 medium aubergine, thinly sliced
2 beef tomatoes, sliced
50 g/2 oz/1 cup diced feta cheese
60 ml/4 tbsp low fat natural (plain) yogurt
olive oil
paprika and garlic salt

1 Sprinkle the aubergine slices with garlic salt, leave for 30 minutes, then rinse and dry.

2 Preheat the oven to 200°C/400°F/Gas 6. Brush a baking dish with olive oil and arrange the aubergine and tomatoes so that they are slightly overlapping. Scatter with feta cheese and spoon over the yogurt.

3 Sprinkle with paprika and garlic salt, then bake for 25–30 minutes, or until bubbling and golden brown. Serve hot.

PRAWNS AND CHICORY IN WALNUT DRESSING

This walnut dressing is surprisingly low in fat – and walnuts are low in saturated fat, too.

Serves: 4   *Preparation time:* 5 minutes

30 ml/2 tbsp chopped walnuts
30 ml/2 tbsp unsweetened apple juice
30 ml/2 tbsp low fat natural (plain) yogurt
1 head chicory
200 g/7 oz peeled cooked prawns
salt and black pepper
watercress sprigs

1 Blend the walnuts, apple juice, and yogurt in a food processor. Alternatively, finely chop the walnuts and stir the ingredients together. Season well.

2 Slice the chicory and arrange with the prawns and watercress on four serving plates. Spoon the dressing over and serve.

FISH

THAI MACKEREL PARCELS

Mackerel is rich in the beneficial fatty acids that reduce fat levels in the blood. This makes it an ideal fish to include in any diet.

Serves: 4   Preparation time: 10 minutes
Cooking time: 15–20 minutes

15 ml/1 tbsp sunflower oil
4 medium mackerel, cut into 8 fillets
60 ml/4 tbsp chopped fresh coriander
2 garlic cloves, thinly sliced
30 ml/2 tbsp finely chopped fresh ginger
finely grated rind and juice of 1 lime
30 ml/2 tbsp light soy sauce

1 Preheat the oven to 180°C/350°F/Gas 4. Place four fillets of fish on large squares of foil.

2 Mix together the coriander, garlic, ginger, and lime rind, then spread over the fish. Top with the remaining fish fillets.

3 Close the foil tightly and place each parcel on a baking sheet. Bake for 15–20 minutes. Mix together the lime juice and soy sauce and spoon over the fish before serving.

POACHED SALMON WITH CITRUS FRUITS

This elegant dish is simple enough for any day of the week.

Serves: 4   Preparation time: 10 minutes
Cooking time: 12–15 minutes

2 shallots, finely chopped
300 ml/$\frac{1}{2}$ pint/1$\frac{1}{4}$ cups fish stock
4 salmon cutlets, about 175 g/6 oz each
1 lime
1 medium orange
1 small pink grapefruit
salt and black pepper

1 Place the shallots in a pan with the fish stock. Simmer gently for 6–8 minutes until the stock has reduced by half and the shallots are transparent.

2 Arrange the salmon on top, then cover and simmer gently for 5 minutes until the salmon are just cooked.

3 Meanwhile, remove a few strips of citrus rind for the garnish, then peel and segment the fruits, collecting the juices.

4 Add the fruit segments and juices to the pan, heat gently, and season to taste. Serve hot or cold.

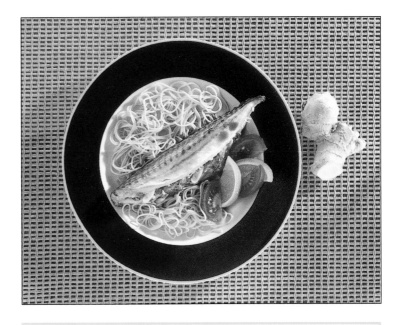

355 CALORIES A PORTION

Oily fish, such as mackerel, herring, sardines, salmon, and trout provide fat-soluble vitamins A and D. Fish oil has been much acclaimed because of its fatty acids, which help make the blood less likely to clot, thereby reducing the risk of heart attack and stroke.

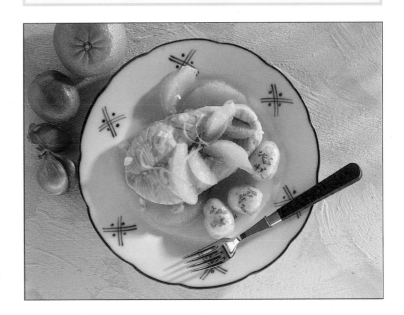

220 CALORIES A PORTION

In light of recommendations to eat less red meat and, in exchange, more fish meals in order to reduce saturated fat in the diet, this is a deliciously healthy, low fat recipe. Combining the fish with citrus fruits is not only unusual but adds lots of Vitamin C to the dish.

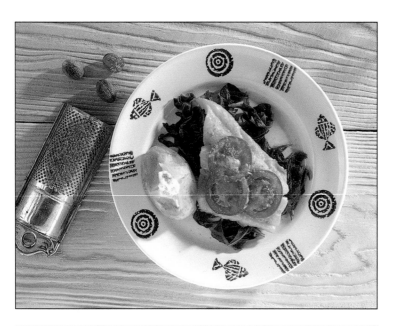

165 CALORIES A PORTION

Spinach is packed with nourishment, providing calcium, iron, vitamins A (as beta-carotene) and C, and fibre. White fish such as cod is high in protein, minerals, and vitamins as well as low in fat, so this makes a scrumptious low-calorie recipe for slimmers.

SMOKED COD AND SPINACH BAKE

If you prefer, unsmoked cod can also be used in this simple dish.

Serves: 4   *Preparation time:* 10 minutes
Cooking time: 25–30 minutes

500 g/1¹/₄ lb fresh spinach
500 g/1¹/₄ lb smoked cod fillet
4 medium tomatoes, sliced
2.5 ml/¹/₂ tsp grated nutmeg
30 ml/2 tbsp grated Parmesan cheese
salt and black pepper

1 Preheat the oven to 200°C/400°F/Gas 6. Wash the spinach, then drain it and cook without water in a covered pan until it has wilted. Drain well and place in an ovenproof dish.

2 Cut the fish into four pieces and arrange them on top of the spinach. Cover with a layer of tomatoes, then sprinkle with nutmeg, Parmesan cheese, and black pepper.

3 Bake for 20–25 minutes, or until the fish flakes easily. Serve hot with jacket or new potatoes.

MONKFISH KEBABS WITH LEMON AND THYME

Oily fish such as mackerel or herring are also good cooked in this way.

Serves: 4   *Preparation time:* 5 minutes
Cooking time: 7–8 minutes

675 g/1¹/₂ lb monkfish
   fillet
15 ml/1 tbsp olive oil
1 garlic clove, crushed
finely grated rind and juice
   of 1 lemon

30 ml/2 tbsp chopped
   fresh thyme
salt and black pepper
lemon wedges

1 Cut the fish into even-sized pieces and place in a medium-sized bowl.

2 Add the olive oil, garlic, lemon rind and juice, thyme, and seasoning, then stir well to coat the fish evenly.

3 Thread the fish pieces on to four wooden skewers and secure with lemon wedges at each end. Cook under a hot grill, or on a barbecue, for 7–8 minutes, turning once.

4 Serve hot with green salad and crusty bread.

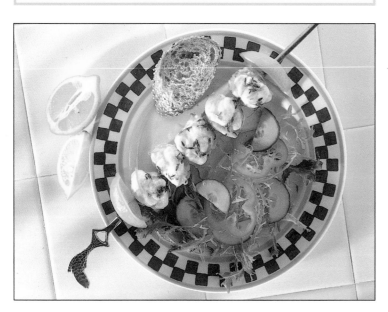

150 CALORIES A PORTION

Another wonderfully low fat, low calorie recipe for slimmers – just watch what you serve it with. Use an oil-free dressing for a side salad and no butter on the bread. Choose freshly baked whole grain bread or one of the many continental varieties, which are so delicious you won't miss the butter.

TAGLIATELLE WITH SMOKED TROUT AND DILL

This light pasta dish can also be made with canned tuna fish or salmon as a quick storecupboard alternative.

Serves: 4   *Preparation time:* 5 minutes
Cooking time: 12–15 minutes

350 g/12 oz tagliatelle
275 g/10 oz smoked trout fillet, skinned
225 g/8 oz cherry tomatoes, halved
150 g/5 oz/^{2}/$_3$ cup low fat natural (plain) fromage frais
   or yogurt
30 ml/2 tbsp chopped fresh dill
30 ml/2 tbsp chopped fresh chives
salt and black pepper

1 Cook the pasta in boiling, lightly salted water until just tender. Drain well.

2 Flake the fish and toss into the hot pasta with the tomatoes and fromage frais or yogurt.

3 Heat gently, without boiling, then stir in the herbs and black pepper. Serve hot.

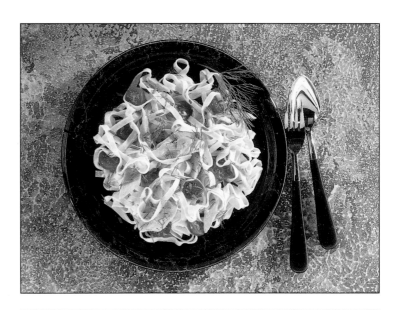

465 CALORIES A PORTION

This recipe at first appears high in calories, but based on pasta, it's nourishing and filling and needs no accompaniment. Use wholemeal pasta for three times more fibre than the white variety. Low fat fromage frais can frequently be used in place of cream in sauces, so consider this low fat option in other recipes too.

GRILLED HALIBUT WITH THAI PEPPER SAUCE

Any other white fish can be used here – try cod or haddock instead.

Serves: 4   *Preparation time:* 15 minutes
Cooking time: about 15 minutes

2 red (bell) peppers, halved and seeded
30 ml/2 tbsp lime juice
5 ml/1 tsp Thai red curry paste
4 halibut cutlets, about 150 g/5 oz each
oil for brushing
salt and black pepper
4 fresh coriander sprigs

1 Place the peppers, skin side up, on a baking sheet. Cook under a hot grill until the skins are blackened. Cover and leave to cool.

2 When cool enough to handle, peel the peppers and place them in a food processor with the lime juice and curry paste. Blend until smooth.

3 Brush the fish lightly with oil, sprinkle with salt and black pepper and grill, turning once, until the fish flakes easily. Garnish with a sprig of coriander and serve on a bed of pepper sauce with accompanying salad.

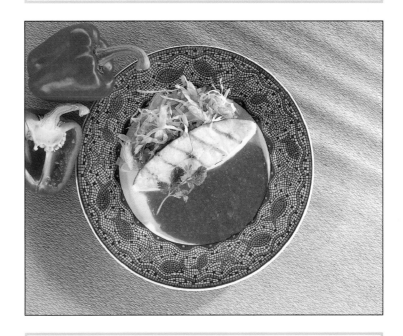

150 CALORIES A PORTION

As illustrated here, oriental-style recipes are an excellent example of how flavourings can be used to produce deliciously light, low fat, low calorie dishes. The red peppers provide a fabulous colour as well as Vitamin C.

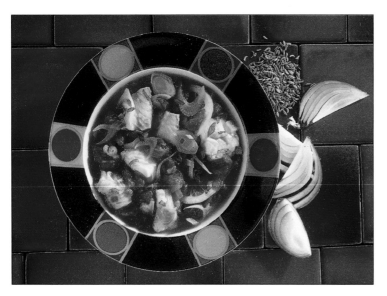

---

135 CALORIES A PORTION

Another example of how we should take ideas from foreign countries, particularly for interesting fish recipes. Many of us tend to eat more meat than fish, and the fish we do eat is frequently fried. Casseroling with vegetables is healthy, low fat, and low calorie.

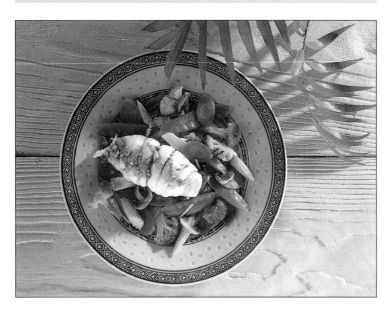

---

265 CALORIES A PORTION

A good selection of vegetables is used in this recipe for a delicious vitamin-packed meal. Stir-frying cooks the vegetables quickly, maintaining their "bite", thus retaining more Vitamin C than if boiled for a longer time in water. The sweetcorn gives added fibre and the mushrooms provide some B vitamins.

ITALIAN FISH STEW

Almost any type of fish can be used for this richly-flavoured main course dish.

Serves: 4   *Preparation time:* 5 minutes
Cooking time: 12–15 minutes

10 ml/2 tsp olive oil	175 ml/6 fl oz /^{3}/4 cup
1 medium red onion, finely	fish stock
chopped	450 g/1 lb cod or haddock
1 garlic clove, crushed	fillet, diced
1 small fennel bulb, sliced	60 ml/4 tbsp chopped
400 g/14 oz can chopped	fresh basil
tomatoes	4 lemon slices
10 ml/2 tsp fennel seeds	salt and black pepper

1 Heat the olive oil in a large pan and fry the onion, garlic, and sliced fennel gently until they are softened but not browned.

2 Add the tomatoes, fennel seeds, and fish stock and bring to the boil. Add the diced fish, basil, lemon slices, salt, and black pepper.

3 Cover and simmer very gently for 6–8 minutes. Serve hot with crusty bread.

CHINESE PLAICE

A wok with a lid is ideal for this recipe, but if you don't have one use a large frying pan with a baking sheet to cover.

Serves: 4   *Preparation time:* 5 minutes
Cooking time: 10–12 minutes

15 ml/1 tbsp sunflower oil	175 g/6 oz button mush-
1 medium carrot, thinly	rooms, sliced
sliced	4 plaice fillets, skinned
175 g/6 oz small broccoli	15 ml/1 tbsp grated fresh
florets	ginger
175 g/6 oz mange-tout	6 spring onions, chopped
6–8 cobs baby sweetcorn,	30 ml/2 tbsp light soy sauce
about 115 g/4 oz	salt and black pepper

1 Heat the oil and stir-fry the carrot, broccoli, mange-tout, and corn for 3 minutes. Add the mushrooms and stir-fry for 2–3 minutes.

2 Roll up the plaice fillets and arrange them on top of the vegetables. Sprinkle with the ginger, onions, soy sauce, salt and black pepper.

3 Cover and simmer for 5–6 minutes. Serve immediately.

MEAT AND POULTRY

PORK AND SAGE KOFTA KEBABS

This tasty, low fat meat dish is ideal for grilling or barbecuing.

Serves: 4   *Preparation time:* 10 minutes
Cooking time: 8–10 minutes

400 g/14 oz lean pork, diced
1 medium onion, chopped
75 g/3 oz/$1^{1}/_{2}$ cups fresh wholemeal breadcrumbs
1 egg white
45 ml/3 tbsp chopped fresh sage
finely grated rind of $^{1}/_{2}$ lemon
15 ml/1 tbsp wholegrain mustard
5 ml/1 tsp oil
salt and black pepper
sage to garnish

1 Place the pork and onion in a food processor and chop finely.

2 Add the breadcrumbs, egg white, and seasoning, and process until the mix binds together.

3 Add the sage and lemon rind. Divide the mixture into 8 parts, and shape on to 8 bamboo skewers. Mix the mustard and oil and brush over the kebabs.

4 Cook under a hot grill for 8–10 minutes, turning occasionally. Garnish with sage and serve with rice.

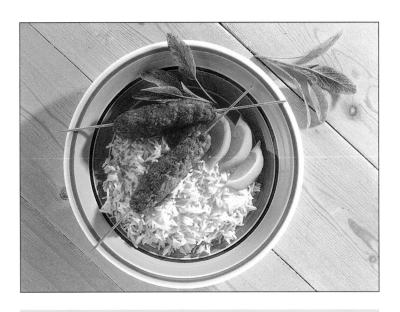

220 CALORIES A PORTION

Meat is a good source of high quality protein, iron, and B vitamins; pork is particularly rich in thiamin (Vitamin B_1). Adding wholemeal breadcrumbs to the minced pork provides fibre. Whenever possible, opt for grilling rather than frying, for healthier, lower fat, lower calorie cooking.

PORK STEAKS WITH PEPPERCORN GLAZE

Nowadays pork is a low fat meat, and is well worth including in a healthy diet.

Serves: 4   *Preparation time:* 5 minutes, plus 30 minutes marinating time   *Cooking time:* 12–15 minutes

4 lean pork loin steaks
15 ml/1 tbsp green peppercorns, crushed
20 ml/4 tsp balsamic vinegar
250 ml/8 fl oz/1 cup stock
4 spring onions, sliced

1 Sprinkle the crushed green peppercorns and the vinegar over the pork, then cover and leave for 30 minutes.

2 Reserve the peppercorn mixture and dry-fry the pork in a heavy or non-stick frying pan until golden, turning once.

3 Add the peppercorn mix, stock, and spring onions, then boil rapidly, uncovered, for 8–10 minutes until the stock has reduced by half and the meat is tender. Serve hot.

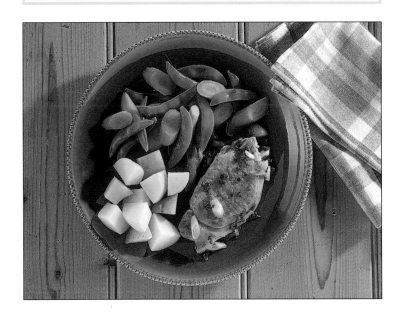

180 CALORIES A PORTION

By using a heavy or non-stick frying pan there's usually no need to add any fat to meat which is simply to be browned in a pan. Even with trimming off any visible fat, there's sufficient fat within the lean tissue to keep the meat moist and prevent it from burning.

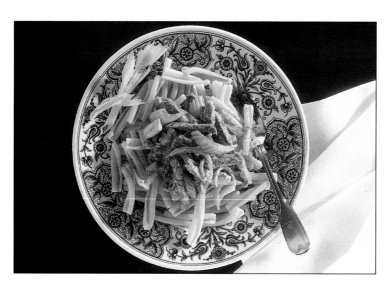

175 CALORIES A PORTION

Although the recommendation is to eat less red meat, choosing lean cuts will significantly reduce your fat intake. Traditionally completed with soured cream, low fat natural yogurt makes a further fat and calorie reduction to the recipe. Although there are some vegetables in this recipe, serve with something green, such as broccoli, for extra Vitamin C.

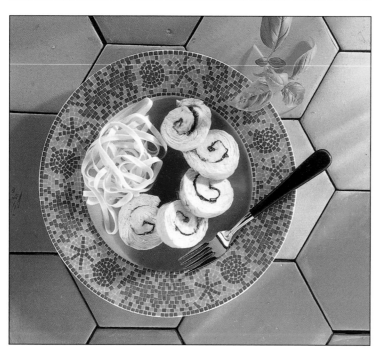

130 CALORIES A PORTION

Turkey makes an excellent choice for very low fat, low calorie meals. It is a lean meat and an excellent source of protein.

BEEF AND CELERY "STROGANOFF"

Choose lean, tender beef, so that it cooks in minutes.

Serves: 4   *Preparation time:* 10 minutes
Cooking time: about 15 minutes

1 small onion, thinly sliced
45 ml/3 tbsp beef stock
450 g/1 lb lean beef sirloin or fillet, cut into thin strips
3 celery sticks, sliced
150 g/5 oz mushrooms, sliced
5 ml/1 tsp cornflour
15 ml/1 tbsp Worcestershire sauce
125 g/4 oz/$\frac{1}{2}$ cup low fat natural (plain) fromage frais or yogurt
salt and black pepper
paprika to garnish

1 Cook the onion and beef stock in a large pan over a moderate heat, stirring until the onion is tender and almost dry.

2 Stir in beef strips and cook over a high heat to seal. Add the celery and mushrooms; cook for 2–3 minutes.

3 Mix the cornflour with the Worcestershire sauce, then stir into the fromage frais or yogurt and add to the meat. Bring to the boil, stirring constantly. Season. Serve with pasta or rice and garnish with paprika.

MEDITERRANEAN TURKEY SPIRALS

Turkey breast steaks have less than 2 per cent fat, and they're very quick to cook.

Serves: 4   *Preparation time:* 10 minutes
Cooking time: 15–20 minutes

4 thin turkey breast steaks
30 ml/2 tbsp red pesto sauce
25 g/1 oz/$\frac{1}{2}$ cup large basil leaves
120 ml/4 fl oz/$\frac{1}{2}$ cup chicken stock
250 ml/8 fl oz/1 cup passata
garlic salt and black pepper

1 Place turkey between two sheets of greaseproof; beat until thin. Spread with pesto sauce.

2 Lay the basil leaves over each steak, then roll them up like Swiss rolls. Secure with cocktail sticks.

3 In a flameproof casserole or large pan, bring the stock and passata to the boil. Add the turkey spirals, cover and simmer for 15–20 minutes or until the juices are clear.

4 Adjust the seasoning and remove the cocktail sticks. Serve hot with pasta or rice and a green vegetable.

SPAGHETTI WITH TURKEY RAGOUT

Turkey mince is much lower in fat than most other meats. Alternatively, look for low fat pork, lamb, or beef mince.

Serves: 4   *Preparation time:* 10 minutes
Cooking time: about 1 hour

450 g/1 lb turkey mince	15 ml/1 tbsp tomato purée
1 medium onion, diced	5 ml/1 tsp dried oregano
1 medium carrot, diced	2 bay leaves
1 celery stick, diced	225 g/8 oz spaghetti
400 g/14 oz can tomatoes	salt and black pepper

1 In a heavy or non-stick pan, dry-fry the turkey mince and onion until lightly coloured. Stir in the carrot and celery and cook, stirring, for 5–8 minutes.

2 Add the tomatoes, tomato purée, dried oregano, and bay leaves, then bring to the boil. Cover and simmer gently for 40 minutes, until tender and reduced.

3 Meanwhile, cook the spaghetti in lightly salted, boiling water until just tender. Drain well, then spoon the ragoût over.

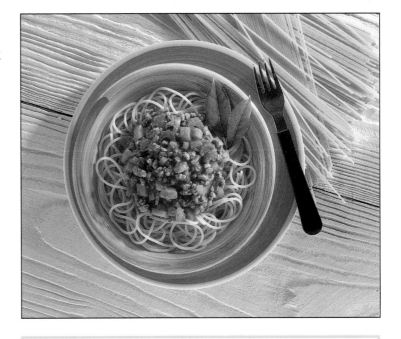

355 CALORIES A PORTION

Using turkey mince rather than beef mince makes a lower fat version of this "bolognese style" recipe. Use wholewheat pasta for added fibre and serve with a fresh green salad for Vitamin C.

SPICY CHICKEN PROVENCALE

This dish is rich in flavours. It is simmered slowly for a highly nutritious meal.

Serves: 4   *Preparation time:* 10 minutes, plus 30 minutes standing time   *Cooking time:* 35–40 minutes

1 medium aubergine, diced	2 garlic cloves, sliced
10 ml/2 tsp olive oil	1 small green chilli, sliced
8 chicken thighs, skinned	2 courgettes, thickly sliced
1 medium red onion, cut into wedges	2 beef tomatoes, cut into wedges
1 green (bell) pepper, thickly sliced	1 bouquet garni
	salt and black pepper

1 Sprinkle the aubergine with salt, then leave to drain for 30 minutes. Rinse and dry.

2 Heat the olive oil in a non-stick pan and fry the chicken until golden. Add the aubergine, onion, pepper, and garlic, and fry gently to soften.

3 Add the chilli, courgettes, tomatoes, herbs, and seasoning. Cover tightly and cook over a low heat for 25–30 minutes until tender.

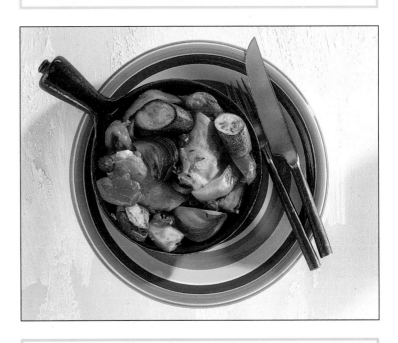

230 CALORIES A PORTION

This "ratatouille style" dish is rich in Vitamin C, supplied by the selection of vegetables. Adding chicken turns it into a more substantial main course meal, and, by skinning the chicken, it remains very low in fat.

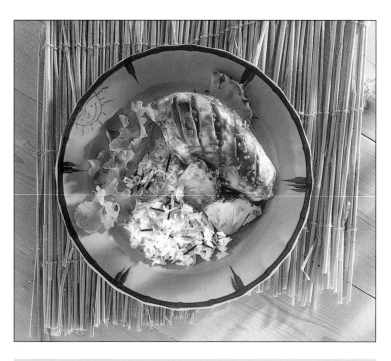

190 CALORIES A PORTION

Adding fruit such as pineapple to a savoury dish is a delicious
alternative to vegetables for packing in some Vitamin C and fibre.

CARIBBEAN GINGER CHICKEN

To save time, unsweetened canned pineapple can be used instead of fresh fruit.

Serves: 4   *Preparation time:* 10 minutes
Cooking time: 30 minutes

4 chicken breasts, skinned	15 ml/1 tbsp dark musco-
1/2 small fresh pineapple,	vado sugar
sliced	15 ml/1 tbsp lime juice
2 spring onions, chopped	5 ml/1 tsp hot pepper
30 ml/2 tbsp chopped	sauce
fresh root ginger	5 ml/1 tsp tomato purée
1 garlic clove, crushed	salt and black pepper

1 Preheat the oven to 200°C/400°F/Gas 6. Slash the
chicken at intervals with a sharp knife. Place in an
ovenproof dish with the pineapple slices.

2 Mix together the onions, ginger, garlic, sugar, lime
juice, pepper sauce, tomato purée, salt and black
pepper. Spread over the chicken.

3 Cover and bake for 30 minutes or until the
chicken juices are clear. Serve with plain and wild
rice and salad.

LAMB TIKKA

The meat for this recipe should be very
lean, so leg of lamb is ideal.

Serves: 4   *Preparation time:* 10 minutes, plus 24 hours
marinating time   *Cooking time:* 15–20 minutes

450 g/1 lb boneless leg of	1 garlic clove, crushed
lamb, cubed	10 ml/2 tsp vinegar
150 g/5 oz/2/3 cup low fat	5 ml/1 tsp chilli powder
natural (plain) yogurt	5 ml/1 tsp turmeric
juice of 1 lemon	5 ml/1 tsp cumin
1 small onion, grated	2.5 ml/1/2 tsp salt

1 Place the lamb in a non-metallic bowl. Mix together
the remaining ingredients and toss with the lamb to
coat it evenly. Cover and chill for 24 hours.

2 Preheat the oven to 220°C/425°F/Gas 7. Arrange the
lamb cubes on a rack in a roasting tin and bake for
15–20 minutes. Alternatively, thread them on to skewers
and cook under a hot grill or on a barbecue.

3 Serve hot, with tomato, cucumber, and mint salad,
yogurt, and grilled papads (poppadums).

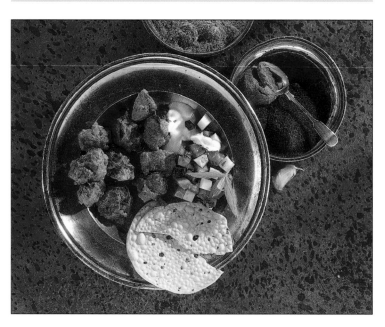

205 CALORIES A PORTION

Use either leg of lamb or lean neck fillets trimmed of fat, rather
than shoulder, which has a higher fat content. The natural yogurt
makes a low fat marinade; grilling or barbecuing keeps the
calories down to a minimum.

VEGETABLES AND SALADS

ROAST POTATO WEDGES WITH GARLIC AND ROSEMARY

A reduced fat alternative to traditional roasties, but just as tasty.

Serves: 4   *Preparation time:* 5 minutes
Cooking time: 35–40 minutes

675 g/1^1/$_2$ lb medium old potatoes
15 ml/1 tbsp olive oil
2 garlic cloves, thinly sliced
60 ml/4 tbsp chopped fresh rosemary
salt and black pepper

1 Preheat the oven to 220°C/425°F/Gas 7. Cut each potato into four wedges and cook in boiling, lightly salted water for 5 minutes. Drain well.

2 Toss the potatoes with the olive oil, garlic, rosemary, and black pepper and tip into a roasting tin.

3 Roast for 30–35 minutes, turning occasionally, until the wedges are crisp and golden brown.

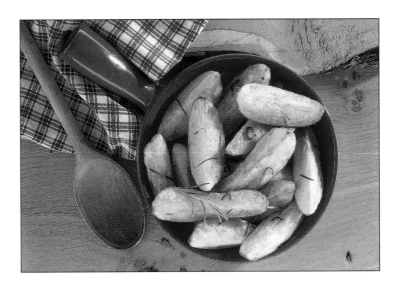

180 CALORIES A PORTION

Potatoes are not particularly high in Vitamin C but because they're eaten in quantity and quite frequently, they do make a significant contribution. Leaving the skins on helps to retain the Vitamin C as well as providing fibre. Garlic is reputed to "clear the blood", lowering blood cholesterol levels and discouraging fatty deposits on the inner walls of the blood vessels.

RED COLESLAW

Red cabbage keeps its crispness very well, so this salad is good for packed lunches and picnics.

Serves: 4   *Preparation time:* 10 minutes

^{1}/$_4$ small red cabbage, shredded
1 small red onion, thinly sliced
4 radishes, thinly sliced
1 red apple, cored and grated
15 ml/1 tbsp red wine vinegar
30 ml/2 tbsp low fat natural (plain) yogurt
5 ml/1 tsp clear honey
salt and black pepper

1 Place the cabbage, onion, radishes, and apple in a wide salad bowl and toss thoroughly.

2 In a screwtopped jar, shake the remaining ingredients until they are evenly blended.

3 Pour the dressing over the salad and toss well. Serve with crusty bread.

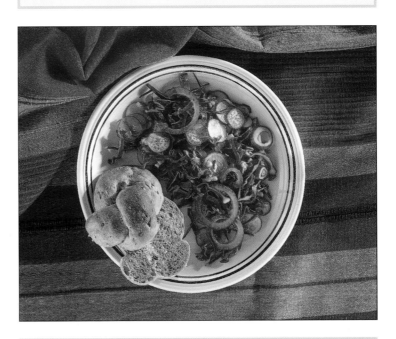

40 CALORIES A PORTION

Red cabbage is rich in Vitamin C and, like all fresh, raw vegetables, retains a higher vitamin content than if it were cooked. The apple and radishes also help boost the vitamin value of this delicious salad.

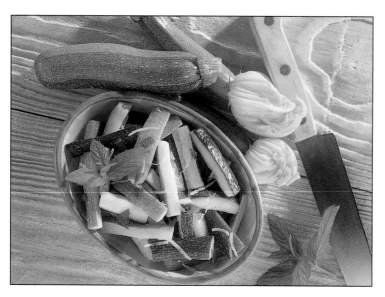

COURGETTES IN MINTED LEMON DRESSING

Courgettes are easy to prepare, and take only minutes to cook.

Serves: 4   *Preparation time:* 5 minutes
Cooking time: 5–6 minutes

450 g/1 lb courgettes
grated rind and juice of 1 small lemon
10 ml/2 tsp low fat spread
45 ml/3 tbsp chopped fresh mint
salt and black pepper

1 Quarter the courgettes and cut them into 6 cm/2$^{1}/2$ in sticks. Place in a heavy or non-stick pan.

2 Add the lemon juice and low fat spread, then cover and cook over a moderate heat, shaking the pan occasionally, for 5–6 minutes until just tender.

3 Add the mint, lemon rind, and seasoning to taste. Serve hot.

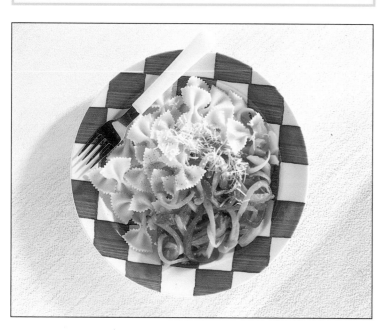

PASTA WITH GRILLED PEPPER SAUCE

This pasta dish is a good vegetarian main course, or it can be served with grilled meats.

Serves: 4   *Preparation time:* 10 minutes
Cooking time: about 25 minutes

4 (bell) peppers, mixed colours, halved and seeded
3 plum tomatoes, peeled and chopped
1 red onion, thinly sliced
1 garlic clove, thinly sliced
350 g/12 oz/6 cups pasta bows or other pasta
salt and black pepper
30 ml/2 tbsp grated Parmesan cheese (optional)

1 Place the peppers, skin side up, on a baking sheet. Cook under a hot grill until the skins are blackened. Cover and leave to cool.

2 Place the tomatoes, onion and garlic in a pan, cover and simmer gently for 8–10 minutes until tender. Peel the peppers and thinly slice. Add to the pan, heat gently and season well.

3 Cook the pasta in boiling, lightly salted water until just tender. Drain well. Toss with the pepper sauce and sprinkle with Parmesan cheese (if using).

SPINACH, APRICOT, AND HAZELNUT SALAD

If you prefer, sunflower seeds can be used instead of flaked hazelnuts.

Serves: 4   *Preparation time:* 5 minutes
Cooking time: 1 minute

75 g/3 oz/2 cups fresh young spinach
75 g/3 oz/$1/2$ cup ready-to-eat dried apricots, chopped
30 ml/2 tbsp flaked hazelnuts
15 ml/1 tbsp sesame seeds
30 ml/2tbsp orange juice
15 ml/1 tbsp balsamic vinegar
30 ml/2 tbsp low fat natural (plain) yogurt
salt and black pepper

1 Place the spinach in a large bowl and toss with the apricots and hazelnuts.

2 In a small pan, heat the sesame seeds gently until they begin to colour and pop. Remove from the heat.

3 Add the orange juice, vinegar, yogurt, and seasoning. Spoon the dressing over the salad and serve with crusty bread.

SUMMER COUSCOUS SALAD

Most couscous is pre-cooked and only needs soaking, so it's a very easy alternative to rice or pasta

Serves: 4   *Preparation time:* 10 minutes, plus 30 minutes soaking time

115 g/4 oz/$1^1/2$ cups couscous
1 celery stick, chopped
$1/2$ small cauliflower, cut into small florets
4 spring onions, chopped
45 ml/3 tbsp chopped fresh parsley
45 ml/3 tbsp chopped fresh mint
15 ml/1 tbsp lemon juice
2.5 ml/$1/2$ tsp chilli sauce
salt and black pepper

1 Place the couscous in a large bowl, cover with plenty of boiling water and leave to stand for 30 minutes. Drain and leave to cool.

2 Stir in the remaining ingredients, season well and toss thoroughly.

3 Spoon into another large bowl or on to a wide platter and serve chilled.

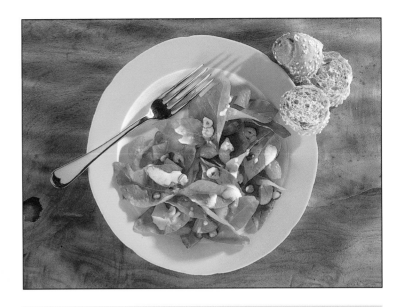

80 CALORIES A PORTION

The dark green leaves of spinach are very rich in Vitamin C. To prepare, tear them rather than cut with a knife so that you preserve as much vitamin content as possible. There's also good supplies of calcium, iron, and Vitamin A (as beta-carotene) provided by the spinach and dried apricots.

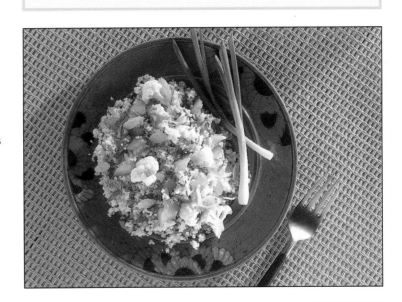

115 CALORIES A PORTION

Couscous is semolina grains coated with wheat flour. Like all cereals it is a starchy carbohydrate food, which we are recommended to eat more of for a healthy diet. If unavailable, bulgar, or cracked wheat, makes a simple substitute since it too only requires soaking. The celery, cauliflower, spring onions, and parsley in this recipe all provide Vitamin C.

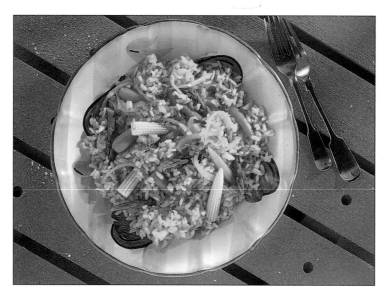

AS A MAIN COURSE FOR 4: 300 CALORIES A PORTION

AS AN ACCOMPANIMENT FOR 6: 200 CALORIES A PORTION

A good variety of different vegetables in this recipe provide plenty of Vitamin C and Vitamin A (as beta-carotene) from the carrots. Rice is a healthy starchy carbohydrate and contains some B vitamins.

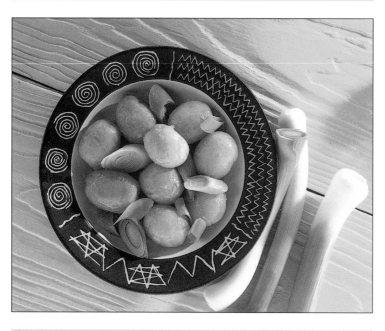

145 CALORIES A PORTION

This is a wonderful low fat method of cooking potatoes, which even slimmers can enjoy. Potatoes play an important part in a healthy diet, as they are an excellent source of starchy carbohydrates and Vitamin C. There is lots of Vitamin C in the leeks as well.

RISOTTO PRIMAVERA

A substantial one-pot vegetarian main dish.

Serves: 4   *Preparation time:* 10 minutes
Cooking time: 25 minutes

250 g/9 oz mixed spring vegetables
10 ml/2 tsp olive oil
1 medium onion, sliced
250 g/9 oz/1 1/4 cups round grain rice
2.5 ml/1/2 tsp ground turmeric
600 ml/1 pint/2 1/2 cups vegetable stock
45 ml/3 tbsp chopped fresh parsley
salt and black pepper
30 ml/2 tbsp grated Parmesan cheese (optional)

1 Leave the vegetables whole if they are small. Heat the oil in a non-stick pan and fry the onion until golden. Stir in the rice and cook 1–2 minutes. Add turmeric, vegetable stock, and seasoning. Bring to the boil, then add the vegetables.

2 Return to the boil, then cover and cook gently, stirring occasionally, for 20 minutes, or until the rice is tender and most of the liquid has been absorbed. Add more stock if necessary. Stir in the parsley, adjust the seasoning to taste. Serve hot, lightly sprinkled with Parmesan cheese (if using).

NEW POTATOES AND LEEKS IN MUSTARD

If you usually crave butter on your new potatoes, try this tasty alternative.

Serves: 4   *Preparation time:* 2 minutes
Cooking time: 15 minutes

500 g/1 1/4 lb small new potatoes
2 young leeks, thickly sliced
120 ml/4 fl oz/1/2 cup stock
15 ml/1 tbsp German mustard
salt and black pepper

1 Cook the potatoes in lightly salted, boiling water for 10-12 minutes or until tender. Drain well.

2 Meanwhile, place the leeks in a separate pan with the stock and mustard, bring to the boil, cover and simmer gently for 5 minutes or until tender.

3 Stir the potatoes into the leeks, adjust seasoning and serve hot.

PUDDINGS AND DESSERTS

PEACHES IN ROSE SYRUP

An easy, elegant summer dessert for any occasion – nectarines or apricots can also be used.

Serves: 4 *Preparation time:* 5 minutes, plus 1 hour chilling time *Cooking time:* 1 minute

8 small peaches
15 ml/1 tbsp icing sugar
10 ml/2 tsp rosewater
a handful of scented rose petals to decorate

1 Plunge the peaches into a large pan of boiling water for 1 minute, then drain and rinse in cold water.

2 Halve and stone the peaches and remove the skins. Arrange in a wide dish and sprinkle with icing sugar and rosewater.

3 Cover and chill for about 1 hour. Decorate with a sprinkling of rose petals and serve with Greek-style yogurt or ricotta cheese.

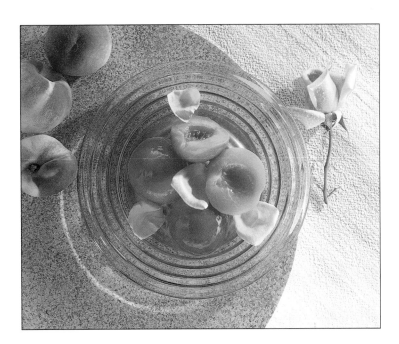

80 CALORIES A PORTION

Peaches provide both Vitamin A (as beta-carotene) and Vitamin C. Adding rosewater to the syrup imparts such a wonderful fragrance and flavour that less sugar is necessary.

BAKED BRAMLEYS WITH BLACKBERRIES

A classic combination of flavours in a healthy, high-fibre dessert.

Serves: 4 *Preparation time:* 5 minutes
Cooking time: 40–45 minutes

4 medium Bramley apples, cored
125 g/4 oz/1 cup fresh or frozen blackberries
15 ml/1 tbsp light muscovado sugar
15 ml/1 tbsp lemon juice
15 ml/1 tbsp low fat spread

1 Preheat the oven to 180°C/350°F/Gas 4. Using a cannelle or sharp knife, cut vertical lines through the apple skin at intervals, then place the apples in an oven-proof dish.

2 Mix the blackberries with the sugar and spoon them into the centres of the apples. Sprinkle with lemon juice and dot with low fat spread.

3 Cover tightly and bake for 40–45 minutes or until the apples are tender. Serve warm with a spoonful of yogurt.

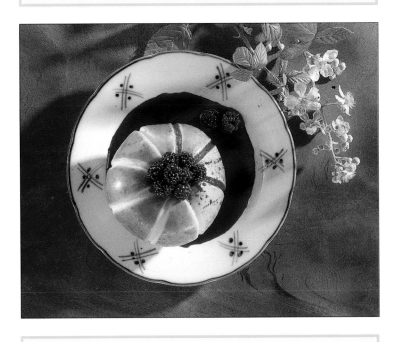

110 CALORIES A PORTION

Lots of Vitamin C and fibre in this recipe are provided by both fruits. Eat the apple skin, which contains fibre. Blackcurrants are a particularly rich source of Vitamin C and could be used in place of the blackberries.

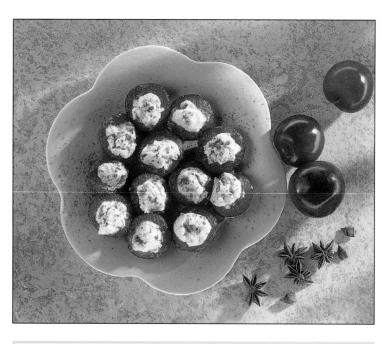

BAKED SPICED PLUMS WITH RICOTTA

Star anise has a warm, rich flavour – if you can't get it, try cinnamon instead.

Serves: 4 *Preparation time:* 5 minutes
Cooking time: 15–20 minutes

450 g/1 lb ripe red plums, halved and stoned
115 g/4 oz/$^1/_2$ cup ricotta cheese or fromage frais
15 ml/1 tbsp caster sugar
2.5 ml/$^1/_2$ tsp ground star anise

1 Preheat the oven to 220°C/425°F/Gas 7. Arrange the plums, cut side up, in a wide ovenproof dish.

2 Using a teaspoon, spoon the ricotta cheese into the hollow of each plum. Sprinkle with sugar and the star anise.

3 Bake for 15–20 minutes, or until the plums are hot and bubbling. Serve warm.

110 CALORIES A PORTION

Plums are not as high in Vitamin C as some other fruits but like all fruit and vegetables they play an important part in a healthy diet. Aim to have at least 4 portions of fruit a day.

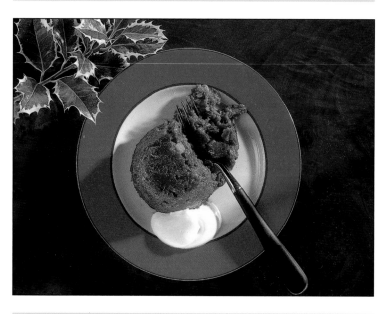

LIGHT LITTLE CHRISTMAS PUDDINGS

Low fat, low sugar, and high fibre, these are much lighter than traditional Christmas puds.

Serves: 6 *Preparation time:* 15 minutes, plus 8–12 hours soaking time *Cooking time:* 2 hours

225 g/8 oz/$^3/_4$ cup mixed dried fruit
juice of 2 medium oranges
45 ml/3 tbsp brandy
1 Bramley apple, grated
1 large carrot, grated
75 g/3 oz/1$^1/_2$ cups fresh wholemeal breadcrumbs
45 ml/3 tbsp plain (all-purpose) wholemeal flour
10 ml/2 tsp ground allspice
45 ml/3 tbsp chopped toasted hazelnuts
1 egg, plus 1 egg white, beaten

1 Place the dried fruit in a bowl and add the orange juice and brandy. Cover and soak overnight. Mix all the remaining ingredients into the fruit.

2 Divide the mixture between 6 lightly oiled 150 ml/$^1/_4$ pint/$^2/_3$ cup pudding cups. Cover with double foil. Steam for 1$^1/_2$ hours; top up the water regularly.

3 Unwrap the puddings and wrap again individually in greaseproof paper and foil. Store for up to 3 weeks. To serve, steam for a further 30 minutes.

210 CALORIES A PORTION

Unlike other fruit, dried fruit does not provide Vitamin C, but it does provide some iron, calcium, fibre, and natural sugar. There's sweetness too in the carrot and therefore there is no need for sugar in this recipe. Using wholemeal breadcrumbs and flour adds fibre to these puddings. Serve with low fat custard or yogurt.

COMPOTE OF DRIED FRUIT WITH CARDAMOM

This richly-scented, satisfying winter fruit compote is rich in fibre.

Serves: 4 *Preparation time:* 5 minutes, plus 8 hours standing time *Cooking time:* 2–3 minutes

1 orange
1 Earl Grey tea bag
6 cardamom pods, lightly crushed
250 g/9 oz/2 cups dried fruit salad

1 Thinly pare the rind from the orange and place it in a large bowl with the tea bag and cardamom. Pour over 600 ml/1 pint/2^{1}/2 cups boiling water. Leave for 5 minutes, then remove the tea bag.

2 Add the dried fruit, then cover and leave to stand for 8 hours, or overnight.

3 Pour the contents of the bowl into a large pan and heat gently until almost boiling. Squeeze the juice from the orange and add it to the pan. Serve warm.

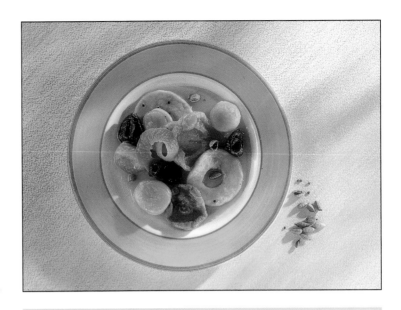

105 CALORIES A PORTION

A high fibre fruit salad. Dried fruit makes a useful store-cupboard alternative for a healthy dessert when few fresh fruits are available. Dried fruit is also naturally very sweet so a sugar syrup is unnecessary, particularly with the perfumed flavour added by the cardamoms.

APPLE AND RASPBERRY CRUMBLE

A high-fibre pudding that's low in added sugar – use honey if you prefer.

Serves 4 Preparation time: 15 minutes
Cooking time: 40–45 minutes

450 g/1 lb Bramley apples, peeled, cored, and sliced
150 g/5 oz/1 cup fresh or frozen raspberries
30 ml/2 tbsp light muscovado sugar
5 ml/1 tsp ground cinnamon
50 g/2 oz/1/2 cup plain (all-purpose) wholemeal flour
50 g/2 oz/1/2 cup plain (all-purpose) flour
50 g/2 oz/2/3 cup porridge oats
50 g/2 oz/4 tbsp soft margarine

1 Preheat the oven to 180°C/350°F/Gas 4. Toss together the apples, raspberries, sugar, and cinnamon and tip into a 1.2 litre/2 pint/5 cup ovenproof dish.

2 Combine the flours and oats in a bowl and mix in the margarine using a fork. Sprinkle evenly over the fruit.

3 Bake for 40–45 minutes until golden brown. Serve warm.

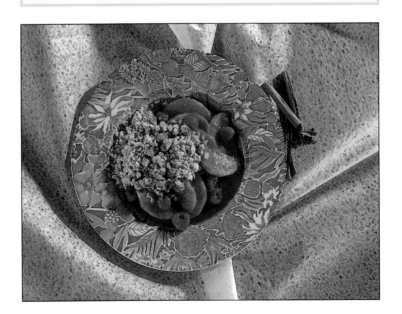

330 CALORIES A PORTION

This is quite a high calorie dessert but provides lots of fibre from the fruit, wholemeal flour, and oats. Raspberries are a good source of Vitamin C. Oats are richly nutritious; they provide B vitamins and minerals and appear to help lower blood cholesterol levels.

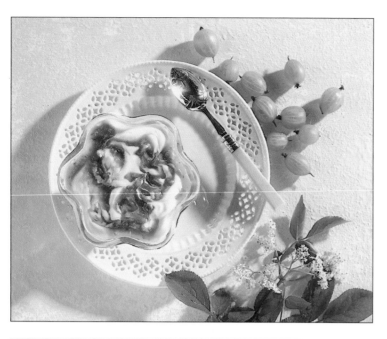

---

130 CALORIES A PORTION

Another low calorie dessert that is rich in Vitamin C from the gooseberries. Greek-style yogurt provides a "creamy" taste and consistency without the high fat and calorific value of cream.

GOOSEBERRY ELDERFLOWER SWIRL

If elderflowers are not available, use a spoonful of elderflower cordial instead.

Serves: 4   *Preparation time:* 5 minutes
Cooking time: 5–8 minutes

350 g/12 oz/3 cups gooseberries
30 ml/2 tbsp caster sugar
2 elderflower heads
250 g/9 oz/1 cup Greek-style yogurt

1 Place the gooseberries, 15 ml/1 tbsp water, and sugar in a heavy pan. Heat gently until the juice runs.

2 Add the elderflowers, then cover and simmer gently for 5–8 minutes, until the gooseberries are tender. Leave to cool.

3 Remove the elderflower stalks and mash the fruit, or purée it in a blender.

4 Place alternate spoonfuls of fruit and yogurt into tall glasses, swirling gently for a marbled effect. Chill until ready to serve.

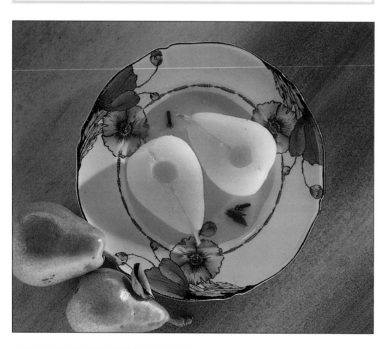

---

90 CALORIES A PORTION

There's Vitamin C from the pears and orange juice and fibre in the pears. No added sugar is necessary with the sweetness from the fruit and cider, making this a delicious low-calorie dessert.

MULLED PEARS IN CIDER

The spices in this recipe make it taste more alcoholic than it really is!

Serves: 4   *Preparation time:* 10 minutes
Cooking time: 25–30 minutes

4 firm, ripe pears, peeled
250 ml/8 fl oz/1 cup sweet cider
150 ml/1/4 pint/²/₃ cup orange juice
thinly pared rind of 1 orange
2 cinnamon sticks
4 cloves

1 Halve the pears and remove the cores. Place the pears in a pan with the cider, orange juice, orange rind, cinnamon, and cloves.

2 Bring to the boil, then reduce the heat. Cover and simmer for 25–30 minutes, turning occasionally, until the pears are tender.

3 Carefully lift the pears into a serving dish. Boil the juices, uncovered, until reduced by half. Strain to remove the orange rind, cinnamon sticks, and cloves, then spoon the juice over the pears. Serve warm or cold.

APPLE GINGER CHEESECAKE

Leaving the skins on apples adds fibre; for a smoother texture, peel them.

Serves: 6   *Preparation time:* 20 minutes

175 g/6 oz/1¹/₂ cups crushed ginger biscuits
60 ml/4 tbsp low fat spread, melted
30 ml/2 tbsp clear honey
2 green eating apples, cored and chopped

250 g/9 oz/1 cup ricotta cheese
150 g/5 oz/²/₃ cup low fat natural (plain) yogurt
1 sachet gelatine
rind and juice of 1 lime
apple slices to decorate

1 Stir together the biscuits and low fat spread. Press into the base and sides of a 24 cm/9¹/₂ in flan tin.

2 Place the apples in a food processor with the cheese, yogurt, and honey. Blend until smooth.

3 Dissolve the gelatine in the lime juice, adding a little water if necessary. Working quickly, stir the gelatine into the cheese mixture and tip it into the biscuit-lined flan tin. Chill until set.

4 Turn the cheesecake out on to a serving plate and decorate with lime rind and apple slices.

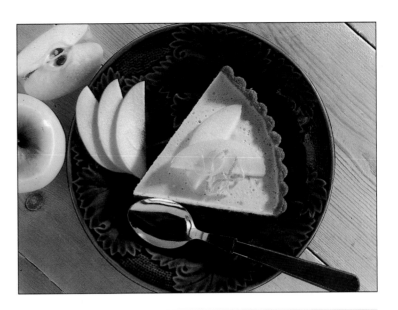

240 CALORIES A PORTION

This recipe is higher in calories than some other desserts, but still significantly lower in fat and calories than most cheese-cakes. The saving is made by using a reduced-fat spread in the base and medium-fat ricotta (or curd) cheese with low fat yogurt for the filling, rather than a high fat cream cheese.

EXOTIC FRUIT SKEWERS WITH MANGO PUREE

Fresh fruit makes the easiest, healthiest dessert you can find – you can choose whatever fruit is in season.

Serves: 4   *Preparation time:* 10 minutes

1 ripe mango, peeled, stoned, and chopped
15 ml/1 tbsp lime juice
¹/₂ small pineapple, cored
1 guava or pawpaw, peeled and seeded
2 kiwi fruit, peeled and quartered

1 Place the mango and lime juice in a food processor and blend until smooth.

2 Cut the pineapple and guava or pawpaw into bite-sized chunks and thread on to four bamboo skewers along with the kiwi fruit.

3 To serve, spoon a little mango purée on to four serving plates and place a skewer on top.

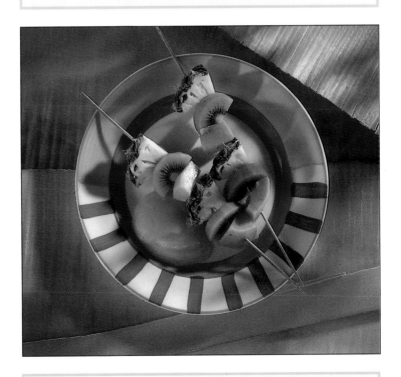

90 CALORIES A PORTION

All these fruits are excellent sources of Vitamin C and served simply like this, you benefit from the maximum value.

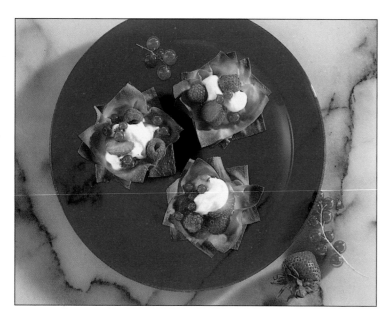

RED FRUITS IN FILO BASKETS

Filo pastry is light as air, low in fat and very easy to use.

Serves: 4   *Preparation time:* 15 minutes
Cooking time: 6–8 minutes

3 sheets filo pastry
10 ml/2 tsp sunflower oil
125 g/4 oz/1 cup mixed
   red summer fruits, such

as raspberries, redcur-
   rants, strawberries
150 g/5 oz/²/3 cup Greek-
   style yogurt

1 Preheat the oven to 200°C/400°F/Gas 6. Lightly brush each sheet of filo pastry with oil, then cut them into 12 pieces, each 10 cm/4 in square.

2 Line 4 small patty tins with three overlapping squares of filo pastry. Bake for 6–8 minutes, until crisp and golden brown. Leave to cool, then turn out on to a wire rack.

3 Reserve a few pieces of fruit for decoration, then stir the remaining fruit into the yogurt. Spoon the yogurt into the filo baskets and decorate with the reserved fruit.

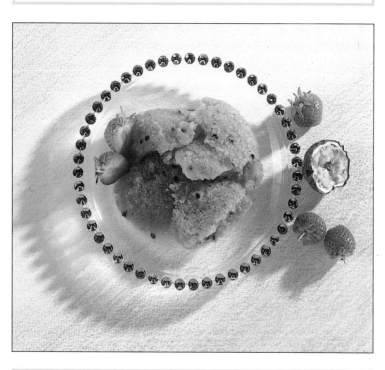

PASSIONATE STRAWBERRY SORBET

Strawberries and passion fruit are naturally quite sweet when ripe, so the added sugar can be kept to a minimum.

Serves: 4   *Preparation time:* 10 minutes, plus freezing time   *Cooking time:* 1 minute

50 g/2 oz/4 tbsp caster sugar
300 ml/1/2 pint/1 1/4 cups water
300 g/11 oz/2 cups ripe strawberries
3 passion fruit, halved

1 Place the sugar and water in a small pan over a low heat and stir until the sugar dissolves. Leave to cool.

2 Purée the strawberries in a blender. Scoop the flesh from the passion fruit and stir it in with the syrup.

3 Pour the mixture into a freezer container and freeze until half-frozen and slushy. Remove from the freezer and whisk hard until the ice crystals have broken up and the mixture is smooth. Freeze until firm.

4 Leave the sorbet at room temperature for 15–20 minutes before serving. Serve with fresh strawberries.

CAKES AND BAKES

LIGHT HONEY AND LEMON SPONGE

Cakes like this one can be included in a diet – but don't eat too many slices!

Makes 1 x 20 cm/8 in cake, 12 slices   Preparation time: 20 minutes   Cooking time: 25–30 minutes

90 g/3^1/$_2$ oz/1 cup plain (all-purpose) wholemeal flour
90 g/3^1/$_2$ oz/1 cup plain (all-purpose) flour
10 ml/2 tsp baking powder
40 g/1^1/$_2$ oz/3 tbsp sunflower margarine
60 ml/4 tbsp clear honey
150 ml/^{1}/$_4$ pint/^{2}/$_3$ cup skimmed milk
finely grated rind of 1 lemon
2 egg whites
45 ml/3 tbsp low-sugar fruit spread
lemon slices and icing sugar to decorate

1 Preheat oven to 200°C/400°F/Gas 6. Line a 20 cm/8 in round, deep cake tin with non-stick paper. Sift together flours and baking powder. Heat the margarine and honey until melted. Stir into the flour with the milk and lemon rind.

2 Whisk egg whites until stiff, fold into mixture. Spoon mixture into the tin, and bake for 20–25 minutes, or until firm. Turn out and leave on a wire rack to cool. Split the sponge in half then sandwich with fruit spread.

SPICED CARROT AND SULTANA LOAF

This high energy, nutritious loaf is great for packed lunches.

Makes: 1 loaf, 12 slices   *Preparation time:* 20 minutes
Cooking time: 40–45 minutes

1 egg yolk, plus 3 egg whites
60 ml/4 tbsp sunflower oil
45 ml/3 tbsp light musco-vado sugar
3 medium carrots, about 225g/8 oz, coarsely grated
75 g/3 oz/^{1}/$_2$ cup sultanas
200 g/7 oz/1^1/$_3$ cups plain (all-purpose) wholemeal flour
5 ml/1 tsp baking powder
10 ml/2 tsp ground allspice
45 ml/3 tbsp skimmed milk

1 Preheat the oven to 180°C/350°F/Gas 4. Line a 21 x 11 cm/8^1/$_2$ x 4^1/$_2$ in loaf tin with non-stick baking paper. Mix together the egg yolk, oil, and sugar.

2 Stir in the carrots and sultanas. Sift the flour, baking powder, and allspice into the mixture, add the flour bran caught in the sieve, and fold in with the milk.

3 Whisk the egg whites until stiff and fold into the mixture. Spoon the mixture into the tin and smooth the surface. Bake for 40–45 minutes, or until firm and golden brown. Cool on a wire rack.

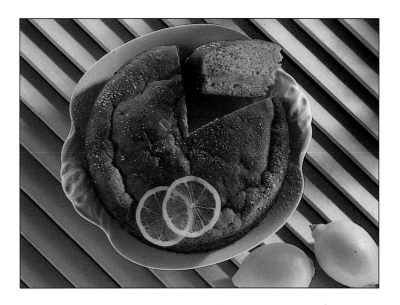

115 CALORIES A SLICE

Using half wholemeal flour increases the fibre content of the sponge without making it heavy. Skimmed milk, rather than whole milk, makes some fat and calorie saving. Low-sugar fruit spreads taste far fruitier than many jams and provide far fewer calories.

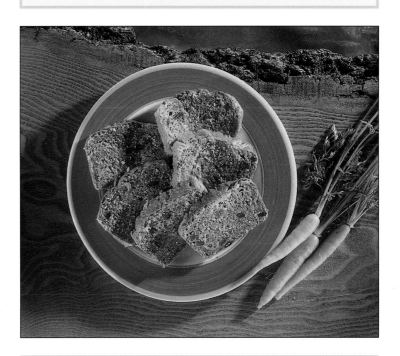

135 CALORIES A SLICE

A high fibre loaf with some natural sweetness provided by the carrots and sultanas. Using wholemeal flour also provides more iron and B Vitamins than refined white flour.

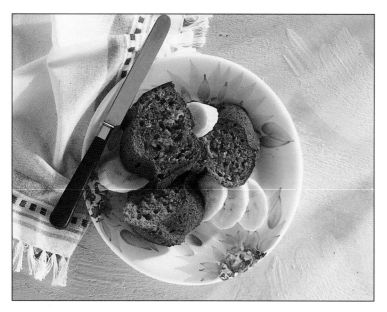

BANANA AND GINGER RING CAKE

Choose really ripe bananas for maximum sweetness.

Makes: 1 ring cake, 14 slices   *Preparation time:* 15 minutes   *Cooking time:* 40–45 minutes

2 size 2 egg whites
50 g/2 oz/1/4 cup light
   muscovado sugar
50 g/2 oz/1/4 cup soft
   margarine
3 ripe bananas, peeled and
   mashed

30 ml/2 tbsp grated fresh
   ginger root
150 g/5 oz/2/3 cup low fat
   natural (plain) yogurt
250 g/9 oz/11/4 cups self-
   raising wholemeal flour
fresh bananas to decorate

1 Preheat the oven to 180°C/350°F/Gas 4. Grease a 23 cm/9 in ring tin. Beat the sugar and margarine until pale.

2 Stir in the bananas, ginger, and yogurt. Fold in the flour. Whisk the egg whites until stiff and fold into the mixture.

3 Spoon the mixture into the tin and smooth the surface. Bake for 40–45 minutes, until firm and golden brown. Turn out on to a wire rack to cool. Decorate with the fresh bananas.

130 CALORIES A SLICE

Wholemeal flour and bananas are high in fibre and makes this cake nourishing as well as filling. Fat is reduced using natural yogurt and egg whites only, and less margarine than more conventional recipes.

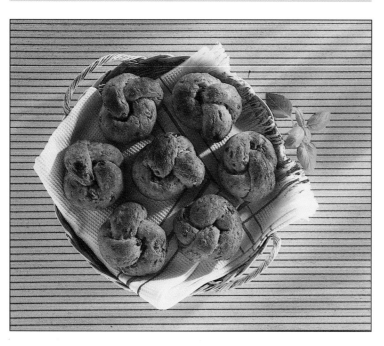

SAVOURY BREAD KNOTS

These simple, low fat bread rolls are flavourful enough to eat without butter.

Makes: 14   *Preparation time:* 15 minutes, plus rising
Cooking time: 12–15 minutes

750 g/11/2 lb/5 cups
   malted brown flour
1 sachet easy-blend yeast
50 g/2 oz/1/2 cup chopped
   sun-dried tomatoes (not
   in oil)

60 ml/4 tbsp chopped
   fresh basil or parsley
450 ml/3/4 pint/17/8 cups
   tepid water
15 ml/1 tbsp olive oil
skimmed milk to glaze
salt and black pepper

1 Place flour, yeast, seasoning, tomatoes, basil, water, and olive oil in a large bowl and mix well. Knead by hand or with a dough hook for 5–10 minutes until smooth.

2 Divide the dough into 14 pieces, roll each piece out like a rope and tie in a knot. Arrange the knots on a greased baking sheet, then cover and leave in a warm place for about 1 hour or until the knots have doubled in size.

3 Meanwhile, preheat the oven to 220°C/425°F/Gas 7. Brush the rolls with milk and bake for 12–15 minutes until well risen and golden brown. Cool on a wire rack.

180 CALORIES EACH

Bread is an important source of starchy carbohydrate, protein, iron, and B vitamins. A healthy diet includes eating plenty of bread – it's just the fat spread on bread which needs reducing.

APRICOT BRAN BREAKFAST MUFFINS

These fruity muffins are more nutritious for breakfast than a slice of toast.

Makes: 12   *Preparation time:* 10 minutes
Cooking time: 15–20 minutes

225 g/8 oz/2 cups self-raising flour
50 g/2 oz/^{1}/$_2$ cup oat or wheat bran
2.5 ml/^{1}/$_2$ tsp bicarbonate of soda
30 ml/2 tbsp soft light brown sugar
115 g/4 oz/1 cup pre-soaked dried apricots, chopped
30 ml/2 tbsp low fat spread
150 g/5 oz/^{2}/$_3$ cup low fat natural (plain) yogurt
200 ml/7 fl oz/^{7}/$_8$ cup skimmed milk

1 Preheat the oven to 220°C/425°F/Gas 7. Mix together the flour, bran, bicarbonate of soda, sugar, and apricots.

2 Melt the low fat spread and add with the yogurt and milk. Mix thoroughly and spoon into 12 greased muffin tins.

3 Bake for 15–20 minutes, then turn out of the tins and serve warm. The muffins are best eaten within 2 days.

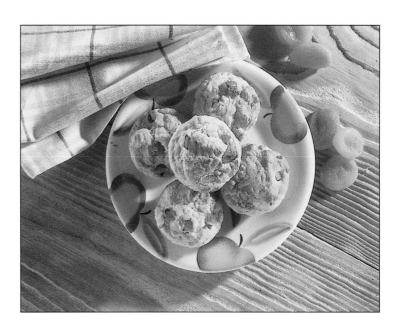

120 CALORIES EACH

Dried apricots add calcium, iron, Vitamin A (as beta-carotene) and some B vitamins to these tasty muffins. Wheat bran provides extra fibre and B vitamins. Using yogurt, skimmed milk, and reduced-fat spread, there's very little fat in the recipe.

APPLENUT COOKIES

These chewy cookies will satisfy a sweet tooth without breaking the rules.

Makes: 14   *Preparation time:* 10 minutes
Cooking time: 12–15 minutes

150 g/5 oz/1^1/$_2$ cups porridge oats
5 ml/1 tsp ground mixed spice
50 g/2 oz/4 tbsp low fat spread
45 ml/3 tbsp demerara sugar
1 eating apple, cored and chopped
45 ml/3 tbsp chopped hazelnuts
1 egg white

1 Preheat the oven to 200°C/400°F/Gas 6. Combine the porridge oats and spice in a bowl and mix in the low fat spread using a fork.

2 Add the sugar, apple, hazelnuts, and egg white, and stir well until the mixture binds together.

3 Form the mixture into 14 small balls; arrange on a baking sheet and flatten the tops slightly.

4 Bake for 12–15 minutes, or until firm and golden brown. Cool on a wire rack. Eat them while still fresh.

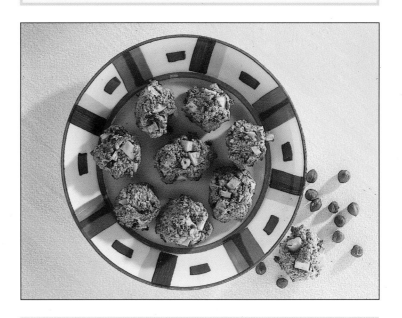

85 CALORIES EACH

Oats are richly nutritious, providing protein, B vitamins, and various minerals. Hazelnuts are lowest in fat, and therefore calories, of all nuts, but add some iron and B Vitamins. The combination of apple and nuts means that both fat and sugar can be reduced, making a tasty, substantial biscuit.

HEAD TO TOE

SOME WOMEN ARE BETTER THAN OTHERS AT INDULGING THEMSELVES, BUT THOSE WHO DO MANAGE TO FIND PAMPERING TIME IN A BUSY DAY OR WEEK ARE USUALLY THE ONES WHO LOOK AND FEEL BETTER ABOUT THEM-SELVES. FINDING TIME FOR SELF-INDULGENCE IS NOT ABOUT HAVING NOTHING BETTER TO DO THAN LIE AROUND ALL DAY DECADENTLY HAVING YOUR HAIR AND NAILS DONE; IT IS ABOUT SELF-PRESERVATION. MOST OF US PUSH OURSELVES TO THE LIMIT IN TERMS OF THE TIME AND ENERGY WE GIVE TO OUR FAMILIES, HOMES, AND CAREERS; SO WE DESERVE TIME ALONE TO RELAX AND RECOUP OUR ENERGY. SNATCH HALF AN HOUR FOR YOUR-SELF IN THE EVENING AND ENJOY IT: TIME SPENT PAMPERING YOUR BODY WILL INSPIRE YOU AND ALLOW YOU TO REACH YOUR SELF-IMPROVING GOALS THAT MUCH FASTER.

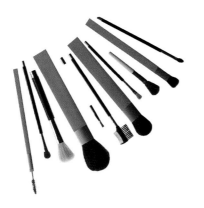

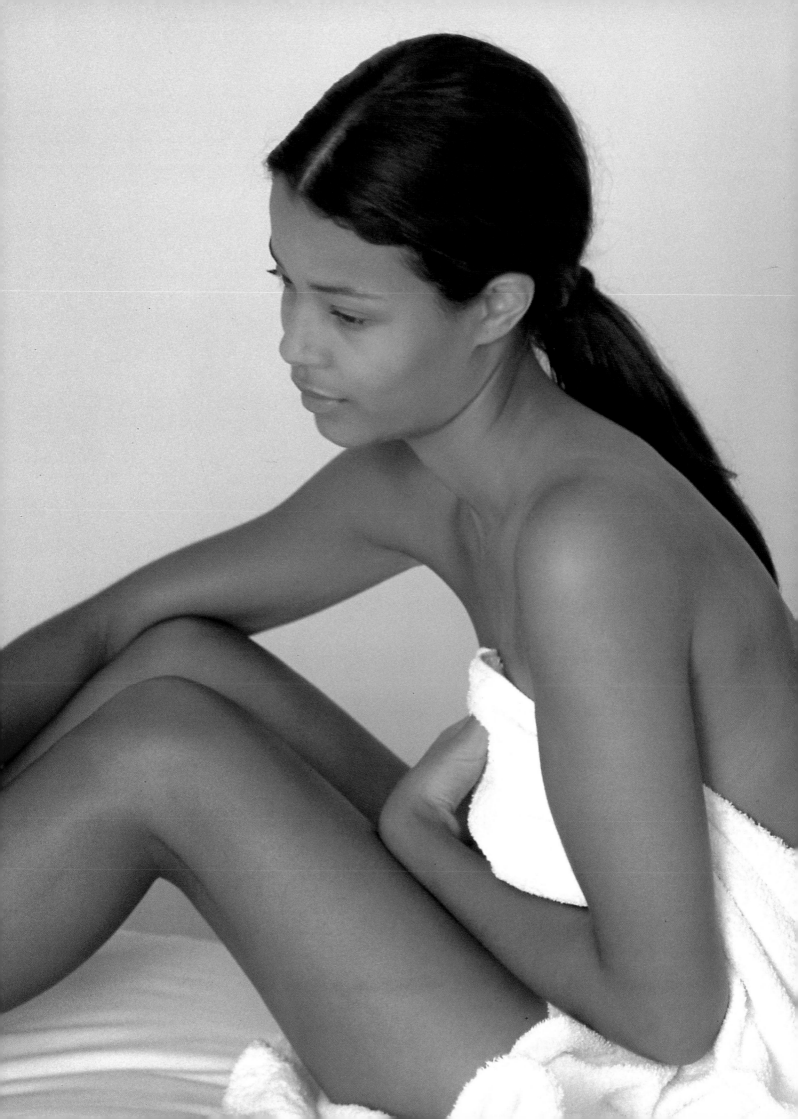

SKIN CARE

Your skin, like your body shape, is inherited. How it behaves, looks, and ages is mainly influenced by your genes, and there is nothing you can do to change this. What you can do, though, is improve its tone, texture, and tendencies, and help delay what the experts call premature ageing by defending it from outside influences such as ultraviolet (UV) light and pollution.

SKIN FACTS

Skin is the body's biggest organ; it insulates us when it is chilly and cools us down with sweat when it is hot. But our skin is much more than a natural thermostat: together with the skeleton, it prevents our internal organs from being damaged by knocks, jolts, and ultraviolet light; its sensory receptors respond to pain, temperature, and touch; and it can nourish, clean, renew, and heal itself. Skin is a multi-functional organ, and it ages faster where it is exposed. Skin on our buttocks, upper back, and inner thighs ages more slowly, probably because it is usually protected by our clothing.

SKIN TYPES

The type of skin you have should determine how you care for it, so it is important to know what your skin type is.

Oily skin produces excess sebum, which makes the face shiny, especially down the central panel – your nose, forehead and chin – where there are lots of sebaceous glands. Oily skin is very often sallow with large pores.

Dry skin can look dull, feels tight after cleansing, and flakes, chaps and wrinkles much more quickly than any other skin type.

An egg and some olive oil make an excellent nourishing and skin-softening face mask when mixed together.

Combination skin is probably the most common skin type; it is oily down the central panel and dry on the cheeks.

Sensitive skin can also be both oily and dry; it is easily disturbed by skin-care products and cosmetics, it tends to go blotchy and tends to have broken veins.

Normal skin is smooth-textured and even-toned with tiny pores.

THE BASICS OF SKIN CARE

Skin care can be confusing these days because there are so many products around. As a guideline, your skin needs two staples: cleanser and moisturizer. Other products – toner, exfoliator, and eye cream or gel – are extras. If you are using more than three or four products daily, and your skin keeps breaking out or reacting, you may be trying too hard. Simplify your routine (it should not take more than 10 minutes to do twice a day), and use basic formulas. You really will be amazed by the speed at which your skin improves.

Cleanse Use water-soluble emulsions or gels (with tepid – not hot – water) or wipe-off lotions. If your skin is oily, use pH-balanced soap-free bars. Splash your face with water – it instantly gives your skin better tone.

DRY SKIN BEATER

An egg and oil mask is suitable for all skin types, in particular dry skin. It is nourishing and softening, and restores sapped tone. Beat a whole egg, add a dash of oil (regular cooking oil will do) and mix in well. To apply, saturate a ball of cotton wool with the mixture and stroke it over exfoliated skin. Leave for a minimum of 10 minutes (you will be able to feel the mask drying) and rinse off using tepid water. Pat your face dry using a soft towel.

Tone If you want to tone, buy alcohol-free toner or use rosewater to freshen your skin. If your skin is dry and you have been using toner, stop and it will instantly improve.

Moisturize Ideally use water-based creams or emulsions; if your skin breaks out a lot, try a lighter, oil-free moisturizer.

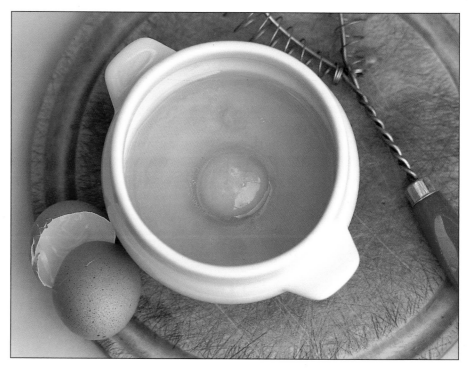

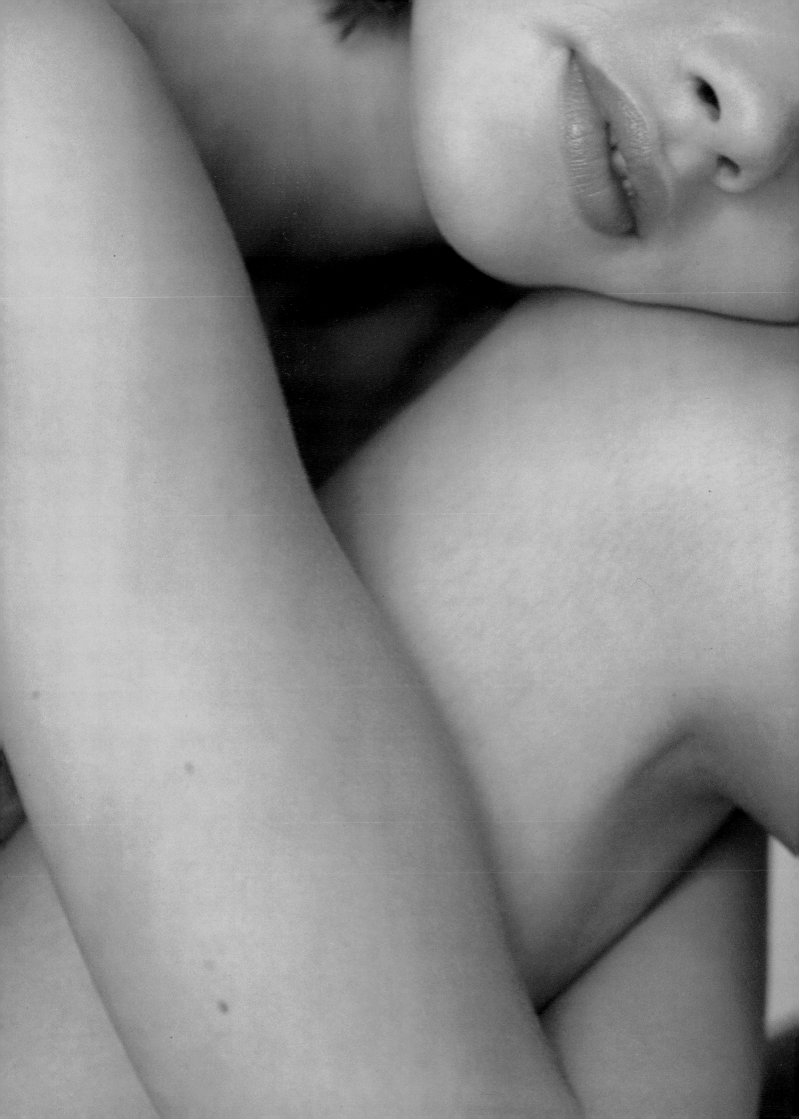

Exfoliate Do this once a week only. Too much buffing over-stimulates and irritates your skin. Fine-grained exfoliators remove dead skin cells and instantly soften your skin.

Mask Simple mud- and clay-based cleansing masks are messy but effective. Rich cold creams make good moisturizing masks for dry or sun-exposed skin: smother your skin with the cream, let the skin

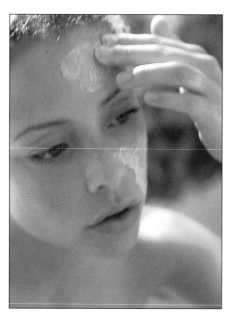

Above and below: Fine-grained exfoliators should be massaged gently into the skin, and then rinsed away thoroughly.

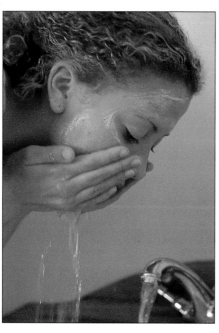

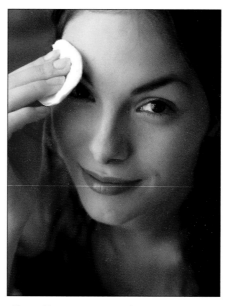

Above: Toners improve skin texture. Apply to oily skin after cleansing

absorb as much of the cream as possible and wipe off the excess with a soft tissue.

OUTBREAK ANSWERS

If your skin has been reacting badly or breaking out, change your skin care products. You may find that you are sensitive to fragrance and certain ingredients. If you have spots, leave them alone – do not squeeze them. When you apply face cream, avoid covering whiteheads with it. If you get blackheads, clean your skin with medicated soap but do not be too

NATURAL NOURISHERS

Aloe vera and avocados are two great natural skin-nourishers; they contain a high proportion of vitamins and minerals, and avocados make excellent face masks for dry skin. They boast 14 minerals as well as the antioxidant vitamins E and A. To prepare a face mask, mash up an avocado, add a touch of sweet almond oil and smooth the mixture over your face; keep it on for as long as possible to make your skin soft.

obsessive about it: skin needs gentle handling.

TIME-DEFYING SOLUTIONS

Our skin begins to age from birth and various changes take place as we get older.

20s to mid-30s Sebaceous and sweat glands are still developing so the skin becomes oily and can suffer from acne or spots. However, it

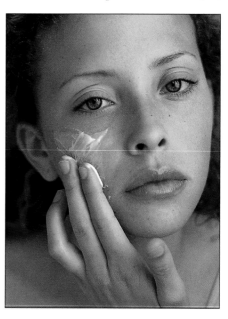

Above: Use upward and outward strokes to apply moisturizer. *Below:* Tap under-eye creams and gels on with your fingertips.

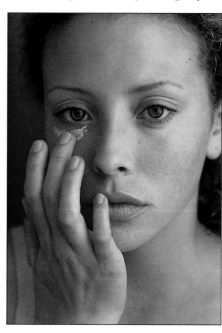

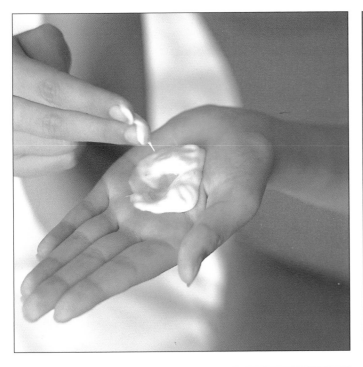

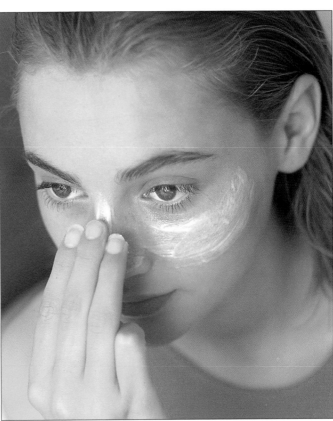

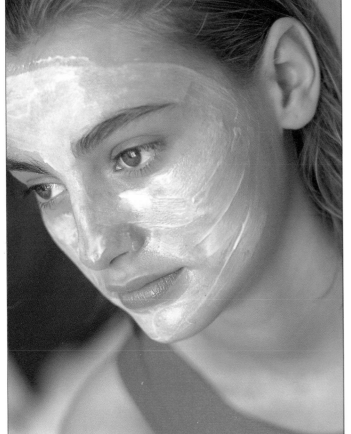

Use cleansing or nourishing face masks at least once a week. *Top:* Put some of the mask into your hand first. *Top right:* Then stroke it over clean exfoliated skin, avoiding the eye area. *Above:* Relax for 10 minutes. *Right:* Rinse the face mask off thoroughly with tepid or warm water.

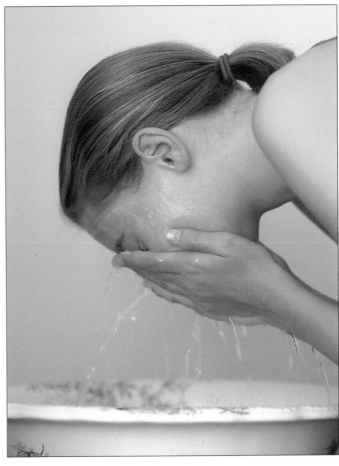

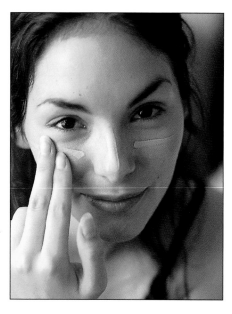

A light moisturizing emulsion is the most suitable type for young skins.

heals fast and has good elasticity, clarity, and tone.

Late 30s Skin colour alters slightly; the tone can be a bit uneven, and the skin is not as springy or elastic; fine lines begin to appear and, because the sebaceous glands have at last settled down, some dryness of the skin can occur.

FIRMING SLACK CHEEK MUSCLES

Fill your mouth up with as much water as possible and hold it there for as long as you can to exercise your muscles: the water pressure does all the work.

40s and older The skin becomes thinner, drier, and more uneven in tone. For those who sunbathed regularly in their youth, years of sun-exposure really begin to take their toll on faces and necks, and lines that already exist may deepen, especially around the eyes and the mouth.

Your skin's needs change as it ages. Tiredness manifests itself more quickly and makes you look pale; regular exfoliation and massage can help to restore the colour. Skin becomes drier with age so it needs a richer (but not heavier) moisturizer and a more gentle cleanser. You can make your own cleanser by mixing 3 drops of essential oil, 1 tsp of cider vinegar,

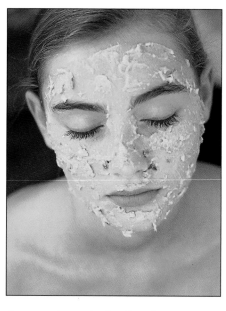

An avocado mashed with a drop or two of olive oil is an excellent skin conditioner.

and 200 ml/7 fl oz bottled or boiled water together. If you are bottling the blend ready for use, use a glass bottle and first sterilize it and its stopper or lid by washing with warm soapy water and then leaving to dry in a low oven for 30 minutes. Sandalwood, vetiver and lemon

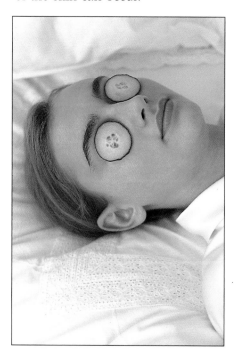

Cucumber slices placed over the eyelids are a natural aid for puffy eyes.

EYES – FOUR FAST DE-PUFFERS

○ Put a teaspoon in the fridge for an hour or overnight, remove it and place the bulb of the spoon over your eye, first making sure it is not too cold or freezing, as this may damage your skin.
○ Soak two cotton wool wedges in chilled rosewater, squeeze out the excess and rest them on your eyes for 20 minutes.
○ Take a couple of slices of cucumber and rest them on your eyes for 20 minutes.
○ Rest for about 15 minutes with two damp tea bags over your eyes; tea bags are said to help fade under-eye bags because they contain tannin and polyphenols which have an astringent effect.

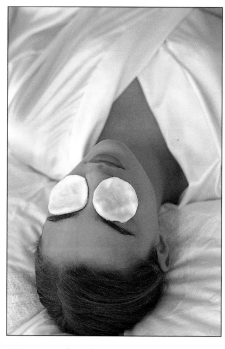

Cotton wool pads soaked in rose water and put over the eyelids soothe tired eyes.

aromatic oils are best for dry skin; frankincense is often recommended for older skin and rose oil usually suits everyone. You can quickly deal with age-related problems using the eye and chin remedies described on the previous page and below.

HOW TO DEAL WITH ACNE

Acne spots are blocked sebaceous glands – basically the same as blackheads and whiteheads, and often inflamed; the problem can occur on your face and also on your back and chest. Hormonal changes are the main cause of acne. The following guidelines can help to improve things. Cleanse your skin twice a day with a light cleansing emulsion only – no toner. Various skin treatments are available for acne-sufferers, but if the problem is severe visit your doctor (who can prescribe a variety of treatments to apply to the skin or to take by mouth). Natural ultraviolet light helps, but because of the health risks linked to UV exposure and sunbeds, it is best not to do this too regularly. Too much ultraviolet light is damaging to the skin so use sunblock creams or lotions if you are outside in hot weather for prolonged periods.

TIPS FOR YOUNGER-LOOKING SKIN

No product can reverse the signs of age; wrinkles are there for good. It is a case of prevention rather than cure, yet you can disguise fine lines with clever make-up and also buy products that temporarily firm your skin, as well as primers that counteract sebum output and make your skin matt and your make-up last longer.

Moisture, however, is the key to young-looking skin: it stops the tissues from becoming dehydrated and creates an automatic barrier against the elements. Some creams

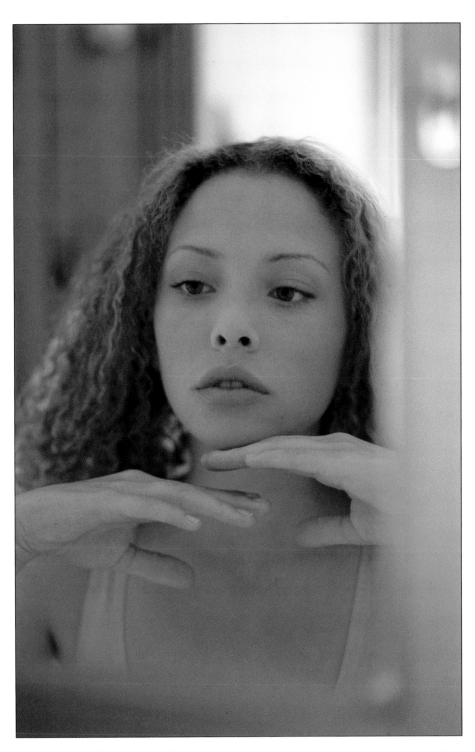

can now feed moisture into your skin and hold it there, temporarily plumping out the tissues. Others improve the texture by exfoliating and moisturizing at the same time. **Moisturizing face masks** Older, drier skin in particular benefits from a nourishing face mask once or twice a week. Add 5 drops of geranium

Using the back of your hands alternately, pat the area beneath your chin, using a quick, stroking-like movement. Do this every day to firm up slack skin and help get rid of a double chin.

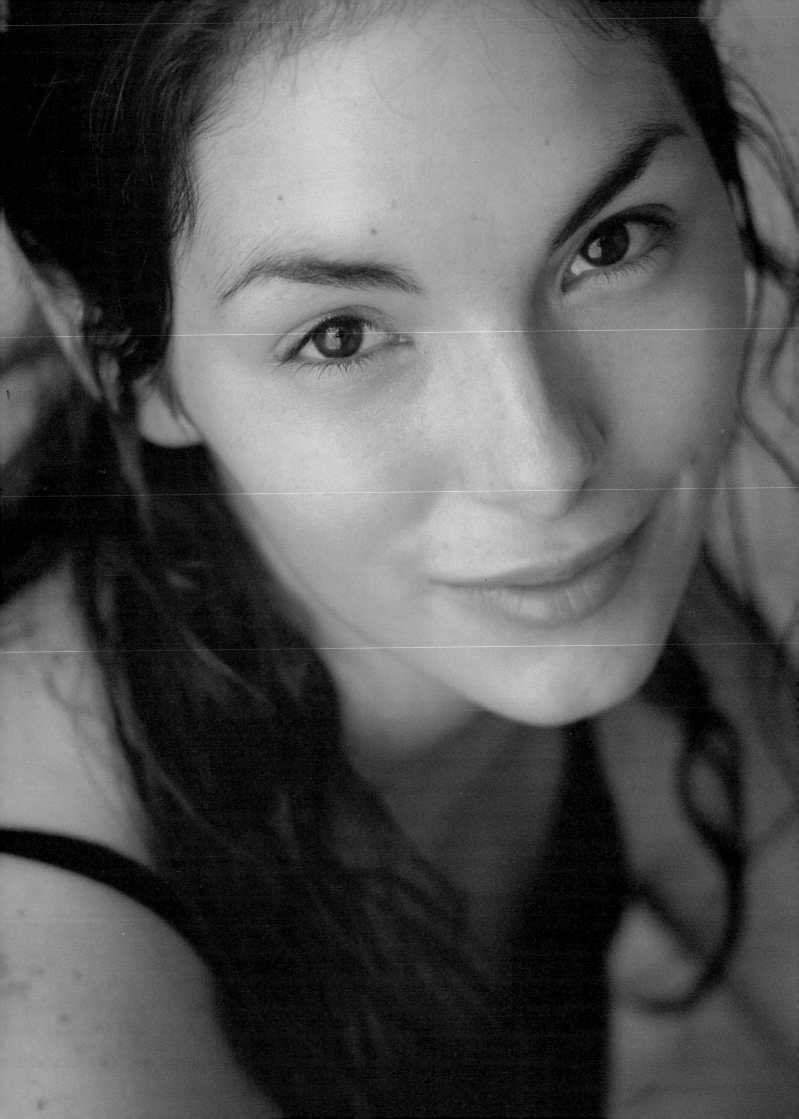

and ylang ylang oil, 8 drops of sandalwood oil and 10 drops of lavender oil to 50 ml/2 fl oz base carrier oil. Gently exfoliate first to remove dead cells and prepare your skin, then apply the aromatic blend using your fingertips. Relax for 10–15 minutes. Wipe off any

---

SUN CARE FACTS

Ultraviolet light, part of the solar spectrum, is now known to be damaging to skin. Most of the UV light that reaches the earth falls into two main wavelength bands: UVA and UVB.

UVA ages your skin; the rays travel far into the skin (they also pass through glass) and start free-radical activity. UVA also increases the cancerous risks of UVB and is responsible for certain skin sensitivity reactions.

UVB burns and browns your skin (by triggering the pigment melanin), and can cause skin cancer. UVB rays are even stronger than UVA.

Infrared light carries the sun's heat to the skin and boosts the effects of the sun's rays.

Tanning is your skin's natural defence mechanism; UV light (mainly UVB) activates melanin, which pigments your skin and turns it darker.

SPF (Sun Protection Factor) shows you the amount of protection a sun cream gives you from UVB rays. The SPF number is a guide to how much time you can stay in the sun before burning, so if you know (from experience) that you can take 10 minutes of sun before beginning to burn, SPF15, for example, allows you 15 x 10 minutes (150 minutes) burn-free sun time.

Star Rating System is a balanced defence rating based on the ratio of a sunscreen's UVA and UVB filters and is shown on the side of sunscreen bottles as a circle of stars; the more stars displayed, the higher the broad spectrum (UVA and UVB) protection.

---

unabsorbed excess using a soft tissue and leave the rest on, ideally overnight.

Atmospheric advice Dry skin usually becomes worse in the winter when central heating saps natural moisture. To remedy this, put a bowl of water near the heat source to increase the humidity.

Stress Make an effort to free yourself from stress; it has a negative effect on your skin, making it pale and drawn.

Broken blood capillaries You do not have to have mature skin to suffer from these; they usually appear on the upper cheeks and although they

---

NATURAL SKIN ELASTICIZERS

Collagen: this gives the skin firmness; collagen contains proteins deep down in the skin, and these weaken with age and exposure to UV light, which is why our skin becomes slacker as we get older.

Elastin: together with collagen, elastin supports our skin and gives it suppleness; with age and exposure, it too degenerates, and cannot be replaced.

---

can be completely masked with make-up they can only be erased surgically. Some preventative actions can help: only use tepid, not hot, water to wash your face, and avoid exposing your face to the sun, especially if your face is unprotected. Always try to apply a sunblock whenever possible.

Liver spots You can buy liver-spot fading creams for your hands.

YOUR SKIN AND THE SUN

When you sunbathe and expose your skin to UV light you damage it for life. The damage does not show up immediately but the sun is the skin's worst enemy: it is the main cause of premature ageing of the skin. If you sunbathed actively in

---

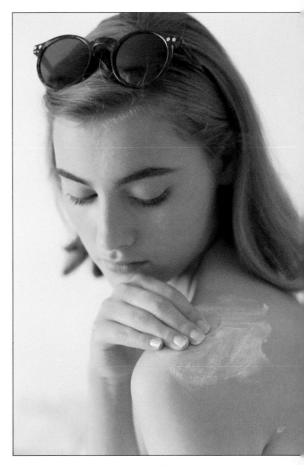

The use of a sunscreen should be an essential part of your skin care routine, particularly in summer and when taking part in winter sports.

FREE RADICALS: SKIN ENEMIES

Free radicals are high-energy molecules in our skin that speed up the ageing process, possibly by damaging collagen and elastin fibres in the skin. Triggered by ageing factors, they get busier as we grow older; however they can be countered with anti oxidants such as C and E vitamins.

---

your 20s the effects – fine lines, wrinkles, loss of elasticity and suppleness, and an uneven texture – would not manifest themselves until you reach your late 30s and early 40s. Pollution, dramatic temperature changes, and harsh detergents can also damage your skin.

BODY CARE

When your mind is fixed on fast improvement it is important to take care of your whole body. For example, rough, mottled skin detracts from an otherwise great figure; but if it's smooth it will improve a not-so-perfect figure – and make a good one look even better.

YOUR BASIC ROUTINE

Include the following steps in your bathroom routine and your skin

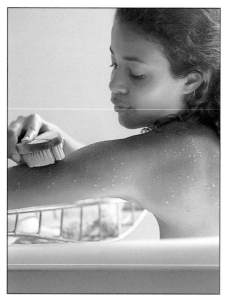

Above: Exfoliate dry areas with coarse-grained scrubs to prepare the skin for moisturizer. *Below:* Oil is nourishing to dry skin.

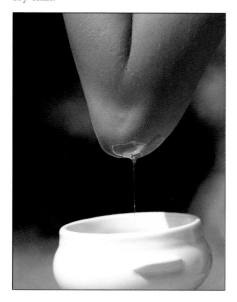

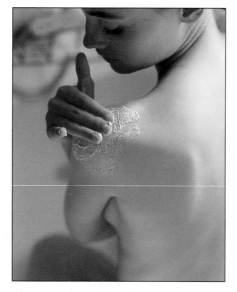

Above and below: Shoulders, upper arms, and elbows in particular benefit from exfoliation.

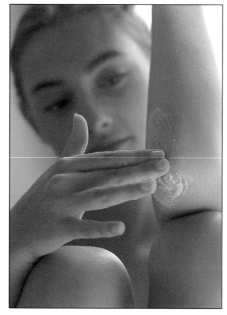

will probably improve dramatically within a few weeks:

Body brush Brushing your skin – from feet to hips and hands to shoulders – with a natural bristle brush exfoliates and tones. You might find that your skin is a bit tender to begin with, but if you use a body brush every day you should be able to build up pressure. After body brushing these areas take time to soak in a warm oily bath to relax.

Exfoliation Body exfoliators have larger grains than facial ones because body skin is tougher. It is easiest to buff in a shower or sauna. Try it – once a week or whenever you have time – on areas that are prone to dry skin, such as your elbows, shins, heels, knees, and your hands.

Moisturizing Pay special attention to thirsty shins, elbows, upper arms, hips, and knees; moisturize when your body is slightly damp and

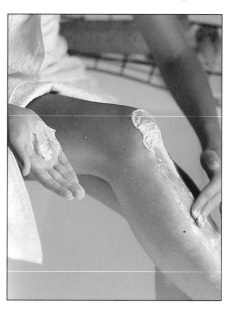

Above and below: After exfoliating, spritz the skin with intermittent bursts of warm and then cool water to boost circulation and skin tone.

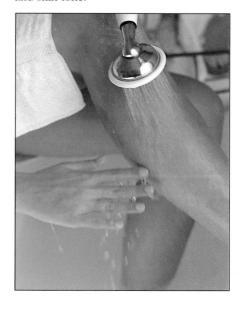

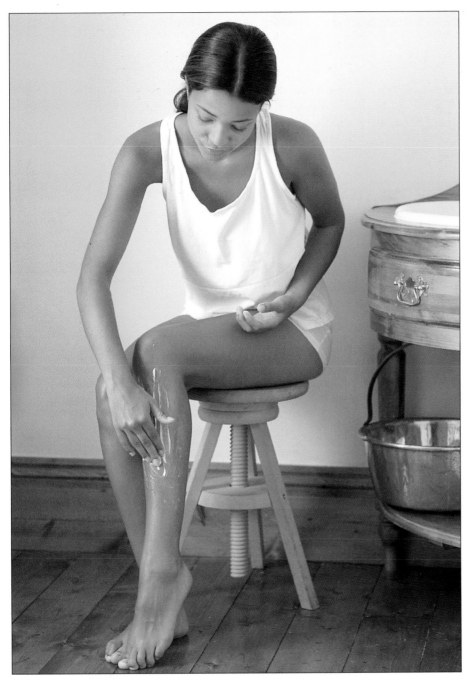

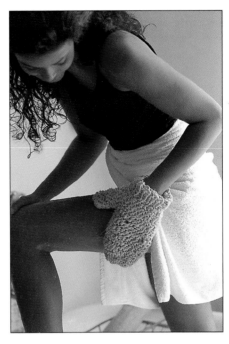

Use a body mitt or body brush every day to smooth skin and pep-up circulation.

○ Spritz your body with cold water; if you can face it after a warm shower, switch to cold and blast your body with chilly water – this is very invigorating.
○ Take exercise – you will be amazed at the warmth regular activity generates.
○ Stop smoking – it hinders your circulation by constricting your blood vessels.

BUST BEAUTY

The average bust is now a size larger than a decade ago; support

Dry areas such as shins and knees need lots of care, especially during the winter when cold weather removes natural moisture from the skin.

warm as creams will sink into the skin much more quickly.

CIRCULATION BOOSTING TIPS

If your toes and fingertips go numb when the weather is not particularly cold, this may be a sign of slow circulation. You may find the following tips helpful:
○ Avoid sitting with your legs crossed. Keep circling your feet at the ankles or pointing and flexing them when you are sitting down. If you have been standing for a long time, slowly rock up and down on your toes for a few minutes.
○ Use a body brush or a rough mitt or loofah; these will help to stimulate your circulation.

STRETCH MARKS

Silvery-grey stretch marks are better prevented than cured. Try using cocoa butter instead of an ordinary body lotion to moisturize problem areas such as your hips, buttocks, thighs, and stomach. Aromatherapy oils are not generally recommended for use during pregnancy, but tangerine essential oil is thought to be a safe stretch-mark reducer for expectant women.

specialists put this growth down to the contraceptive pill, better diet, and increased exercise. There are various topical breast-firming treatments available, but the best way to lift your bust's profile is to exercise the pectoral muscles and diet if you are overweight.

SELF MASSAGE

Regular professional massage is a real treat when you are in the middle of a shape-up plan, it gives you a weekly goal and something to look forward to. If you do not have time to go to a salon, you can do your own massage at home.

HAIR-FREE ZONES

Unwanted excess body hair can cause a lack of self-confidence. A razor is best for removing underarm hair, but there are various options for your legs and bikini line:

Shaving is the quickest and easiest method; stubble will appear within a day or two.

Depilatory creams dissolve hair at the root; regrowth starts within a week.

Waxing, sugaring, and epilators pull hair out at the root; regrowth takes longer, usually a month to six weeks, and the new hairs are often softer than the old ones.

Electrolysis is the only method of permanent hair removal, but it is quite time consuming and expensive; it can also be painful.

AROMATIC REMEDIES

Aromatherapy is an ancient form of alternative medicine that was first practised by Chinese and Egyptian cultures. It has recently been revived as a popular remedial practice. We benefit from aromatherapy through the smell and absorption of essential oils derived from natural substances; the oils are used in massage, as compresses, as skin treatments, in the bath, and as air vaporizers. There are hundreds of oils, each with different qualities, and certain ones can be blended together so that they can offer a number of different benefits. Aromatherapy oils are not recommended for internal use (or during pregnancy) without professional

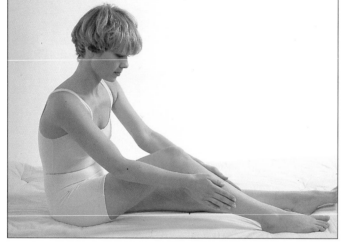

1 Sitting down, lightly stroke oil or moisturizing emulsion on to your legs moving upwards from ankle to thigh; repeat the action from top to bottom five or six times.

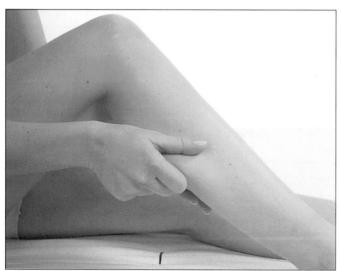

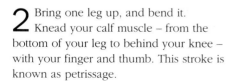

2 Bring one leg up, and bend it. Knead your calf muscle – from the bottom of your leg to behind your knee – with your finger and thumb. This stroke is known as petrissage.

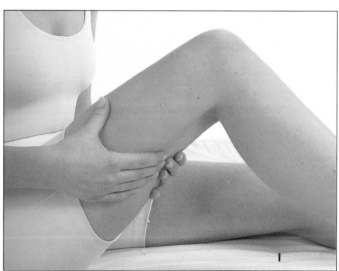

3 Using the same stroke, continue kneading the thigh, working over the top and outside. Then use some smoothing strokes up the back of the leg from ankle to hip.

guidance. Essential oils should only be used in small quantities, and should never be applied directly to the skin – always mix them with a base carrier oil such as sweet almond, safflower, peachnut, or oil of evening primrose.

FAST TONE BOOSTER

Aromatic Massage: a five-minute face massage can revitalize your skin tone. Exfoliate first; while the grains remove dead skin cells the abrasive action brings a rosy glow to the skin. Mix the following aromatic oils with 50 ml/2 fl oz of base carrier oil:

❍ 5 drops of geranium
❍ 5 drops of jasmine
❍ 15 drops of lavender

First warm a few drops of aromatic blend in the palms of your hands, then apply it by cupping your hands over your cheeks and holding them there for a while. Close your eyes, take a deep breath and exhale. Gently rub the oil into your skin in a circular motion using the palms of your hands; massage

ESSENTIAL THERAPIES

Aromatherapy Oil	Benefits
Lavender	Antiseptic, anti-depressant, healing; relieves stress and insomnia, soothes insect bites
Rose	Anti-depressant, aphrodisiac, tonic; helpful for menstrual disorders; aids sleep
Bergamot	Antiseptic, astringent, stimulative; helps to combat oily skin but can sensitize it to UV light
Sandalwood	Healing, antiseptic; can relieve fluid retention, cystitis and insomnia
Patchouli	Healing, soothing; helps combat dandruff and dry skin patches
Ylang Ylang	Antiseptic, aphrodisiac, tonic
Myrrh	Healing, antiseptic, calming; can ease viral and fungal infections such as thrush (if added to a bath)
Juniper	Diuretic, antiseptic, cleansing, calming; avoid in first five months of pregnancy; not to be used by those with kidney disease
Neroli	Calming; soothes nerves and upset stomachs; a good remedy for dry skin
Chamomile, Roman	The most soothing essential oil: relieves anxiety, stress, allergies, and PMS
Geranium	Uplifting and cleansing; astringent, healing
Basil	Reviving, decongestive
Rosemary	Antiseptic, stimulating, balancing; diuretic, uplifting; not to be used in the first 5 months of pregnancy, or by those with high blood pressure
Frankincense	Decongestive, relaxing; aids sleep

AROMATIC SPOT REMEDIES

These aromatherapy blends are ideal for spotty and greasy skins. Add the essential oils to 50 ml/2 fl oz of base carrier oil (such as sweet almond), mix well and massage into your skin; do not rinse as, ideally, the oils should stay on your skin overnight. Use:

❍ 12 drops of cypress*
❍ 12 drops of lemon
or:
❍ 5 drops of cypress*
❍ 5 drops juniper
❍ 12 drops of bergamot
*Avoid using if you suffer from high blood pressure.

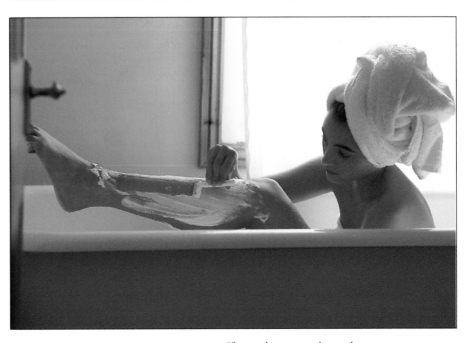

If you shave your legs, always use a cream or gel to soothe and protect your skin. For good grooming, ensure that you shave regularly.

your cheeks then move your hands up to rub smaller circles on your temples; do the same on your forehead and then move down again to your cheeks, and move along your jawline. Using your fingertips, tap gently on the skin below your eyes, moving out across your cheekbones and your temples.

WATER THERAPIES

Relaxing in a bath after a long day is a real treat. It is also very therapeutic as it eases muscle strains and stiff joints, not to mention the benefits it offers your skin and senses if you add nourishing oils, water-soluble milks (Cleopatra preferred the real thing, neat), a herbal bag (hung under a running tap), or a few drops of an essential oil. Bath water should be warm – if it is too hot it can be dehydrating and very exhausting.

Today natural ingredients such as clay, mud, seaweed, and sea salt are often used in professional hydro and thalasso beauty therapies. In hydrotherapy water is used to support the body and provide resistance for the muscles to work against; thalassotherapy is based on sea water and sea derived products, such as seaweeds, salt, and mud.

STEAM CLEANING

Saunas and steam baths are a good way of improving your skin and shedding fluid; you may like to take a body exfoliator into a sauna with you and use it to massage your whole body. Steam rooms, cabinets, and saunas also have a relaxing effect on the body and increase the circulation. Aim to spend 10-15 minutes in the steam room or sauna followed by a cold shower and a 10-minute rest period. Weight-loss treatments, which involve being caked in clay or slimming gels –

and sometimes wrapped in bandages – also work on the principle of fast fluid loss. Most stimulate by means of electrical currents, and incorporate deep-cleansing clay, slimming gels, and bandages. They help your body to release a quantity of fluid, making you feel much thinner instantly, so they are a great boost to your confidence when you are trying to shape-up quickly on a diet and exercise programme.

EARTHY BENEFITS

❍ Clay is naturally astringent, absorbent, and deep-cleansing; it works best as a mask treatment, drawing impurities out and feeding minerals into the skin.
❍ Mud is usually applied as a poultice to ease arthritis, but can also be used to improve the skin
❍ Seaweed is packed with skin-conditioning vitamins, minerals, and trace elements; it is a popular beauty product.

VEIN HELP

Thread veins, wiggly purple lines, usually crop up on the face (around your nostrils or on your upper cheeks) and on your legs. Varicose veins usually occur on your legs; and spider naevi (very small blood vessels in the shape of a spider's web) tend to appear on the upper half of your torso. They can be removed if necessary, although it should be mentioned that, apart from varicose veins, these blemishes are harmless, and even varicose veins do not necessarily need treatment. Options include:
Laser The most modern method, laser beams are used to cauterize broken blood vessels.
Electrolysis Traditionally used for

broken blood vessels on the face, the method cauterizes the veins using a fine needle and electrical current; it can take several attempts before an improvement is seen, and the area can become scabby before it improves. If you choose this method, find a skilled operator.
Sclerotherapy Instead of cauterization, this technique involves injecting a chemical into the blood vessels to seal them so that they no longer receive blood and eventually disappear. Again, it can take several attempts before there is any improvement, but the usual time periods are six weeks for leg veins and three weeks for facial veins.

FAKE TAN – AN INSTANT FIGURE IMPROVER

One of the main reasons why we sunbathe is because we know that a tan makes us look thinner; the knock-on effect of this is increased self-confidence, which is a help when you are baring what you may not consider to be the perfect body in a bikini. The disadvantage is that UV light eventually gives you wrinkled skin, and can cause skin cancer. The next best thing is a fake tan, and the products for these have improved enormously in recent years: they no longer streak or smell; rather they look amazingly realistic and will do wonders for your silhouette. To apply them to best effect follow these guidelines:
❍ Exfoliate to remove any rough skin patches.
❍ Apply the fake tan lotion.
❍ Wipe over heavily creased areas such as your knees, heels, and elbows with damp cotton wool to prevent colour from collecting in the creases.
❍ Allow the tanning treatment at least an hour to settle on your skin before you dress or get into bed.

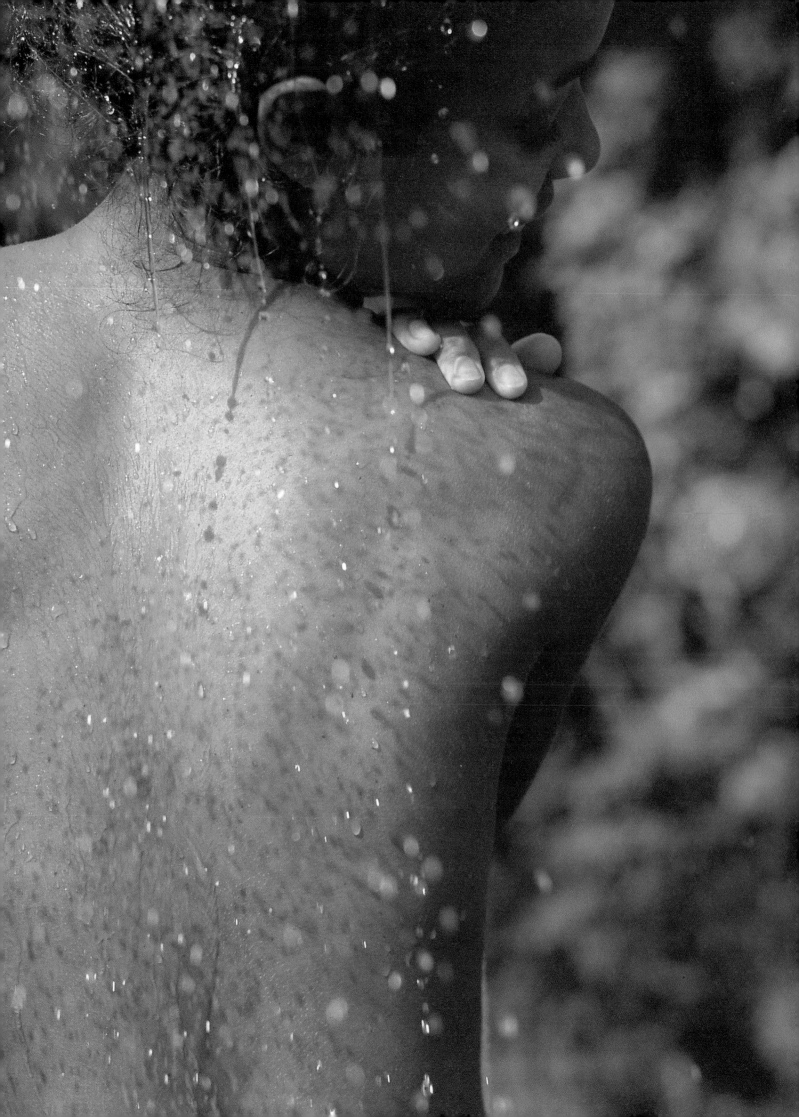

HAIR CARE

Most of us wear our hair the same way for years without changing it. We adopt styles that are practical, and are reluctant to make any great changes because of the fear that they will be wrong or that we will not know how to re-create or maintain the look that has been created by a professional hair-dresser. A cut and colour change can be a real tonic, however, especially if you are after a new look; the trick is to opt for a style that works with – not against – your hair's natural growth pattern and texture.

HAIR BASICS

Your hair's basic needs are cleanser and conditioner, but the type of product you should use depends on your hair type:

Greasy hair can look lank and needs frequent washing with a mild shampoo.

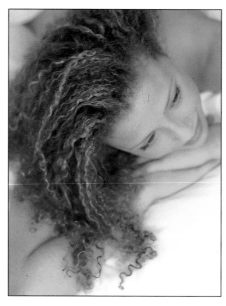

Healthy shiny hair not only looks great, it also reflects good physical well-being and conscientious maintenance.

Dry hair can break easily because it lacks the elasticity of oily or normal hair; it also needs regular washing with a mild but creamy shampoo, and a conditioner.

Normal hair is neither dry nor oily so it does not require any special products unless you wash it frequently, in which case you should choose a gentle shampoo.

Mixed condition hair is oily (normally at the roots) and dry at the ends; it can have split ends and needs care-ful attention with specific products.

HOME-MADE HAIR CONDITIONERS

Healthy hair stretches up to 35 per cent of its length before snapping off; dry hair breaks more quickly because it does not have much elasticity. If your hair feels dry and looks dull, try one of these condi-tioning recipes:

1 Aromatic aid: combine the following oils in 50 ml/2 fl oz of base carrier oil and 10 ml/2 tsp jojoba oil:

○ 10 drops of rosewood oil
○ 5 drops of geranium oil
○ 5 drops of sandalwood oil
○ 5 drops of lavender oil

Apply the mixture to the ends of your hair and leave it on for at least half an hour before washing and rinsing thoroughly.

2 Kitchen cure: boil a handful of ground sesame seeds in a little water for 10 minutes, strain, cool, and apply the mixture to your hair to boost shine, suppleness, and softness.

INJECTING VOLUME

You can achieve root lift and extra volume with styling mousse (which is often lighter than gel) and your hair dryer. Apply the mousse to the roots of hair that is almost dry; tip your head upside down and blast it with the dryer; spray with a setting mist, flip your hair back and spray it once more.

HAIR FAIR?

It is amazing what a difference even the softest tint can make to

---

HAIR COLOURING CHOICES

○ Permanent colour particles change your natural pigmentation by penetrating the hair cuticle; if you are going lighter, hydrogen peroxide is applied to strip the colour out of your hair before it is replaced with chemical dye. The effects last for up to six weeks before you have to have the roots re-done.

○ Semi-permanent colour particles lodge into the cuticle layer but no further. Ideal for Afro, and Asian hair, semi-permanents tend to fade after five or six washes.

○ Tone-on-tone colour is quite a new idea; the basic principle is that it lasts longer than semi-permanent but not as long as permanent colour.

○ Temporary rinses coat the strands with colour; they are not absorbed by the cuticle, are very subtle, good for grey hair, and last for only one wash.

○ Vegetable dyes do not lighten your hair, they simply enhance colour, depth, and shine.

---

your hairstyle, your face and over-all image. If you do decide to take the plunge, go for a shade that complements your skin tone so that it looks realistic. Choose the sort of colour – semi-permanent, perma-nent, tone-on-tone, or temporary – that is easy to maintain. Most hair-dressers now advise going no further than a couple of shades away (darker or lighter) from your natural colour; this is a sound approach because it minimizes the risks of making a mistake and ensures successful results: very often the subtlest changes are the most dramatic.

If your hair is grey or greying, you may choose to high or lowlight it, completely colour it, or let it go. With lights, you can either make your hair look as if it is just begin-ning to go grey or is just a lighter

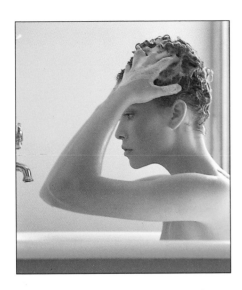

Above: If you wash your hair regularly, use a mild shampoo. *Below:* Always rinse thoroughly with warm water.

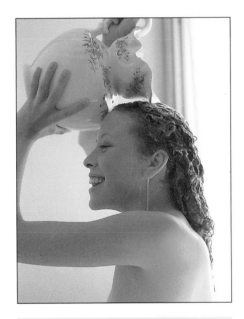

DAILY CONDITIONING?

Whatever you hear or read in advertisements, your hair does not need to be conditioned every day, and that includes conditioning shampoos. Like your skin, your hair has the ability to condition and protect itself, so even if you buy a light, water-based conditioner you only need to use it, at the most, a couple of times a week on the ends of normal hair, and maybe three times a week on dry hair.

Right: Condition when and where your hair needs it, not just for the sake of it.

colour than it really is; with complete colour you can mask grey entirely.

HEAD FOR A CUT AND RESTYLE

This is strongly recommended as a morale-booster, but keep the following two points in mind when you go off for a cut and re-style. First, your hairdresser will know whether the style you choose is going to suit your face. The main thing is to be happy with the style and not choose it because it is fashionable or because everyone else is having it done.

Second, will you be able to keep the style you choose the way it should be? Will it need a lot of fiddling with? If so, think carefully; the most successful haircuts are the ones that are easy to look after.

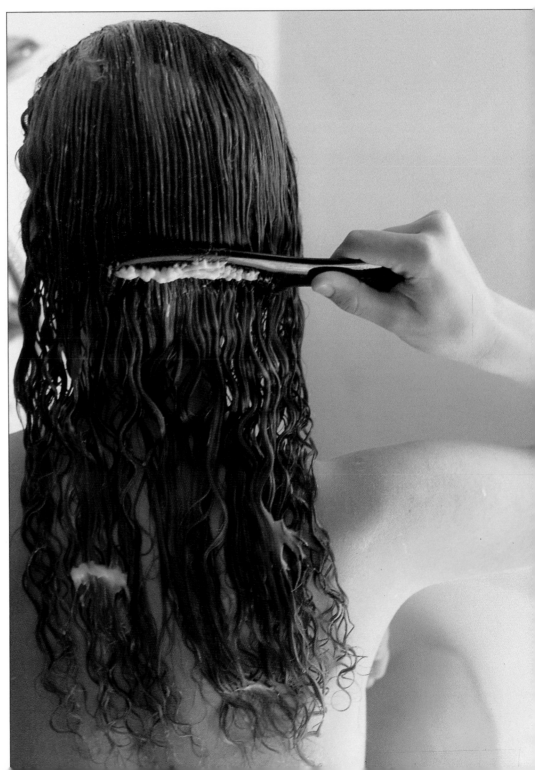

HAND CARE

Hands are always on show, so the ideal is to have smooth skin and nicely manicured nails. But the reality is more usually chapped, dry skin, chipped polish, and broken nails. Our hands are constantly exposed to the elements,

LEMON CLEAN

Bleach stained hands naturally using fresh lemon juice; wash them afterwards with mild unscented soap, and use a pumice stone to remove rough skin; then rub in lots of rich hand cream.

to harsh detergents, soaps, and hot washing-up water. This exposure causes the skin on the backs of our hands to age quickly; liver spots – pigmentation marks that look like oversized freckles – can appear, but these can be lightened with fading creams. To keep the skin on your hands supple, have a bottle of hand lotion by the kitchen sink and, if you dislike wearing rubber gloves, smother your

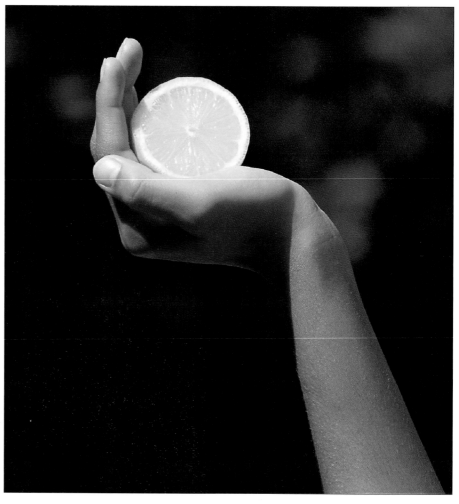

The juice of a fresh lemon is a good natural bleach for both hands and nails.

hands with it before putting them into washing-up water or doing any other kind of housework.

SUPER-SUPPLE SKIN BOOSTERS

Manicurists treat hands that are dry to the point of cracking and callousing with skin-softening warm paraffin wax – the skin is coated with it and then peeled off when set. You can renourish really dry hands at home by soaking them in warm olive oil. Fill a teacup with the warmed oil, dip in your fingers and let them soak for a few minutes. When you remove them, rub the oil into your hands and allow as much of it as possible to be

absorbed before rinsing off any excess. Alternatively, smother your hands with rich cold cream, and pull on a pair of cotton gloves – the heat helps improve the absorption of the cream.

HOME MANICURE

Regular manicures (and a balanced diet) make fingernails strong. Professional manicures are a treat, but you can give yourself a manicure at home without going to unnecessary expense.
○ Use a soft emery board to file your nails, in one direction only, in a shape that suits your fingers – and your lifestyle: pointed talons don't always suit typists or busy mothers.

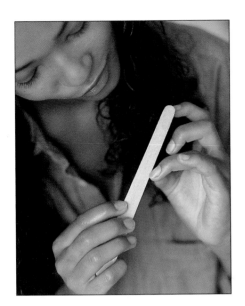

Fingernails should be filed regularly. To minimize breakage, file them straight across with a soft emery board.

The strongest nails are of medium length, filed flat across the top with rounded corners that do not catch.

○ Dip your fingertips in a cup of warm olive oil to soften the nails; if nails are supple, they are less likely to snap off.

○ Rinse and dry your hands; use an orange stick to remove any dirt from underneath your nails.

○ Massage in hand cream; wipe any excess from your nails and apply a base coat of nail polish.

○ Add a coat of coloured or neutral polish on top; allow it to dry, and add a second coat. Apply a top coat to seal the polish and stop it from chipping; keep a bottle of this handy, so that if you are wearing coloured polish you can keep applying it to maintain the colour.

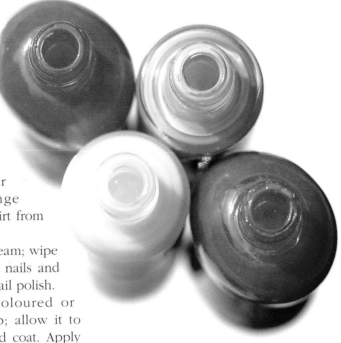

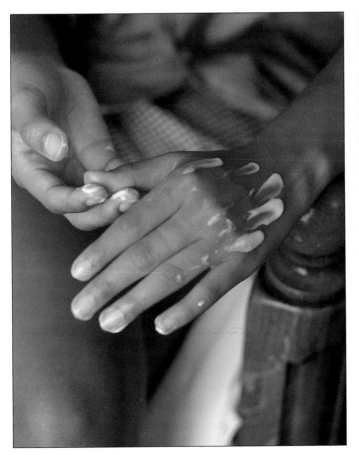

Gently massage hand cream into your hands, remembering to rub it into the skin around the nails. Remove excess with a tissue.

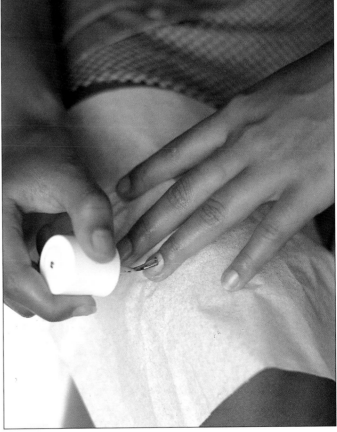

Apply a base coat before putting on coloured or neutral nail polish. Wait for the first coat to dry before applying the second.

FOOT CARE

Most of us do not give our feet the attention they deserve: when they hit the ground they absorb nearly five times our body weight; each foot has 26 bones – a quarter of all the bones in your body – and an intricate network of muscles and tendons. Yet our feet are normally squashed into shoes that do not fit properly (the root of most foot problems), so it is hardly surprising that they feel like a couple of aching blocks at the end of the day.

TIDY TOES

If you look after your feet – keeping toe nails trimmed, removing rough skin, and massaging feet and ankles regularly – you should not have any problems. This simple foot-care routine does not take long – enjoy it a couple of times a week:

❍ Remove any hard skin with a pumice stone or sloughing cream. If you use a foot file rub your skin

---

RELIEVING TIRED AND SWOLLEN FEET

❍ Rest your feet above your head for 10 minutes: do this by lying at right angles to a wall, or on your bed with your feet up on the headboard, or on the floor with your feet resting on the edge of a chair. Any swelling will disappear as trapped fluids travel back up your legs towards your heart.
❍ Plunge your feet into a tub of cold water or sit on the side of the bath with your feet under the cold tap; then put them up for a while.
❍ Roll your feet over a couple of chilled cans of drink straight from the fridge.
❍ Spritz them with a cooling foot spray: you can buy minty ones in most chemists – keep them in the fridge in hot weather.

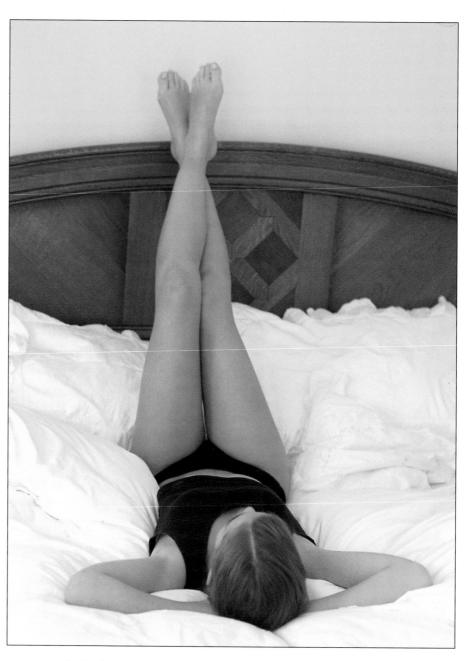

very gently before rinsing off the flaky residue.
❍ Soak your feet for a minimum of five minutes in a bowl or tub of warm water to which you have added some mineral salts or plain sea salt. Bubbling foot spas are a good treat for feet; add a couple of drops of lavender essential oil to soothe aches and ease swelling.
❍ Dry your feet well, especially between your toes; trim your toe-nails by cutting straight across the tip (but not down the sides) and file

Relieve tired and swollen feet by lying with your feet propped up on a bed-head, wall, or chair.

sharp corners with an emery board.
❍ Massage your feet by cupping your hands on either side of your foot and, using your thumbs, firmly pressing the upper part of your foot while pushing your thumbs outwards. Grasp each ankle and gently massage the ankle bone in circular movements to ease away any stiffness.

❍ Wipe any excess grease off your nails and stick tufts of cotton wool between your toes to keep them separate.

❍ Apply a base coat of nail polish, and either leave it at that or cover with coloured polish; when you apply polish start in the middle of the nail with one quick stroke and then work outwards.

❍ Wait for the first coat to dry before applying the next one. Wait for at least half an hour before putting your shoes on.

FOOT PROBLEMS

Feet have a large number of sweat glands, which is why they can smell. Avoiding plastic shoes and keeping them really clean can help, but if you suffer from particularly smelly feet, try wiping surgical spirit over your soles after washing them as this keeps odour at bay. Make sure that you dry your feet well after washing them – fungal and viral infections such as athlete's foot thrive in damp, dark zones.

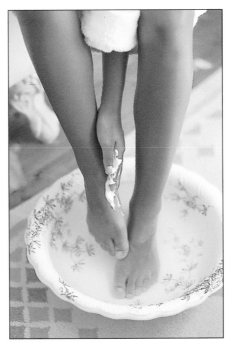

To soften and remove dry skin, first soak your feet in warm soapy water and then use a foot file to remove the dry skin.

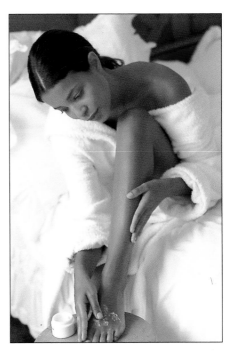

After you have gently filed your feet with a foot file, smooth on foot cream to nourish and further soften the skin.

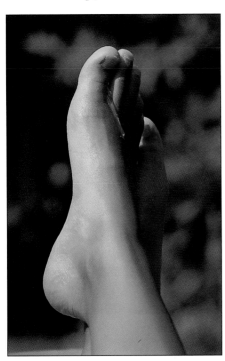

Keep the skin on your feet nourished and smooth with softening oils or creams.

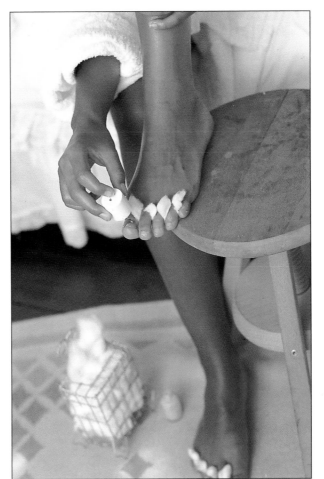

CORN CURES

Never try to tackle a corn yourself with a foot file, but go to see a chiropodist. Soaking your feet in warm soapy water will help to soften corns, and padded rings – which you can buy from most chemists – will ease the pressure.

Wipe the excess cream from your toenails before you apply polish to them.

MAKE-UP

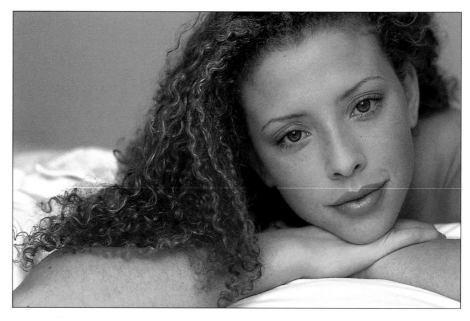

Many women are wary of cosmetics because they are not sure which colours suit them or which make-up methods and textures are the most flattering. Good make-up hinges on experience: you learn what suits you by trial and error. Nobody wants to waste money on a lipstick that turns out to be the wrong colour when you try it at home; but it's very easy to get stuck in a rut – so be brave and experiment a little. Unbiased advice is rare because the cosmetics industry thrives on competitive sales figures. So, it pays to do some research of your own to gain the knowledge that gives you the confidence to choose the cosmetics suitable for you.

HOW TO REASSESS YOUR IMAGE

Take a look at your make-up bag or drawer. How old are the cosmetics in it? Six months, a year – or more? Now study your face when

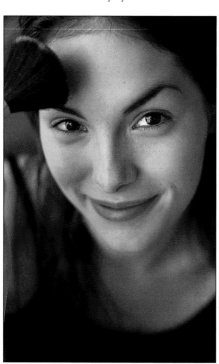

Make-up should be fun to apply, especially when you want to change the way you look.

you are wearing your usual make-up, and ask yourself what it does for you: does it widen or narrow your eyes or mouth, enhance the shape of your face, make you look younger or older? If it does not produce the effect you want and your cosmetics are more than a year old, it is time for a change. Bear these points in mind:

○ **Your age** Make-up that suited you when you were 25 is not going to look right 10 years down the line. Changes in skin tone and texture, as well as in hair colour, require different make-up shades and textures; the right make-up can take years off your face.

○ **Your face shape and skin tone** Make-up can improve face shape by illusion; it can also improve skin tone and texture.

○ **Your eye colour and size** Deftly applied make-up can make small eyes look bigger, blue eyes look bluer and round eyes look longer; can your current make-up do this for you?

○ **Your hair colour** Make-up should complement hair; if your hair is jet black and your skin is pale, deep red lipstick and black eye make-up (mascara and kohl) look stunning;

When applied skillfully, make-up enhances good features and detracts from the not-so-good. With practice anyone can achieve a natural look.

if you are blonde, earthy tones look best (the bright colours can be a bit brassy); if you have brown or black hair you will have almost limitless colour freedom.

○ **Your lifestyle** Make make-up easy; there is no point choosing make-up that requires a great deal of time to apply properly if you have a very busy lifestyle.

A PERFECT COMPLEXION

Do not ignore foundation because you are afraid it will make you look over made-up; because of demand, face bases are now so sheer that you cannot even see them on the skin. Easiest to use are tinted moisturizers, which are just like regular face cream but with added colour. Compact foundations are also easy to apply: these are a mixture of cream colour and powder. Fluid foundations often now have tiny light-reflective grains in them to enhance the look of older skin.

One important point to remember about foundation is that you need to revise the shade in the summer and winter because your skin tone changes colour; it is much paler in winter than in the summer. You can buy shade adjusters to dilute or deepen face bases; one quick way to lighten fluid foundation is to mix it with your moisturizer, and apply the two together like tinted face cream. There are a variety of face bases to choose from:

○ **Fluid or liquid foundations** Today these give fairly sheer coverage; some are also called treatment fluids because they contain moisturizers, UV filters, and skin-firming ingredients. The superior ones have a slip agent in them that helps the fluid glide on to your skin much more smoothly.

○ **Tinted moisturizers** These are face creams that contain colour. They also impart a sheer, natural-looking finish and suit all skin types, especially young skin.

BASE SECRETS

How to apply foundation and how to make it last.
○ Apply it to cool skin as otherwise it melts; hold a cold, damp flannel to your face for a few minutes, dab the skin dry and moisturize.
○ Use matt bases on young skin as they cling for longer; more mature skins benefit from a primer, which makes the complexion matt before any make-up is applied.
○ Apply fluid foundation with your fingers and blend it in well.
○ Let the foundation settle, then dust loose powder on to your nose, forehead, and chin to set the base.

○ **Compact foundations** These are often called "two-in-ones" because they are a blend of cream colour and powder. They are applied with a sponge and usually give fine matt coverage making extra powder redundant.

○ **Foundation sticks** These look like thick lipsticks; you dot them on to your chin, forehead, and cheeks, and then blend the colour on to your skin with your fingers.

○ **Mousse foundation** These are not so common because they are expensive to produce, but they give the sheerest coverage of all, are very easy to apply, and work particularly well for oily skin.

○ **Face tints** These are made up of a water-based coloured-pigment suspension; if you apply them using cotton wool, face tints make it easy to monitor the depth of colour of the foundation layer.

○ **Pastel corrective bases** These are geared to reduce high colour and blotchiness. Mint green and pale blue calm redness (dot them on to your chest too if it gets flushed), pinky-mauve eases yellowy undertones, and apricot warms pale skin.

EYE SHADES
You can own as many as you like, but no one needs to wear three eyeshadows at the same time; two shades – a base and a defining tone – are enough. When it comes to choosing the right colours, professional make-up artists follow these basic rules:

○ **Blue eyes:** all the metallics – gold, bronze, silver, and silver greys; mauve, brown, pink, and fleshy tones.

○ **Brown eyes:** gold, bronze, khaki, pewter, navy blue, mauve, pink, and fleshy tones.

○ **Green eyes:** gold, bronze, grey, earthy tones, fleshy tones.

EYE SHAPE SECRETS
If you have small eyes, never apply liner to the inner rims; put it above or below the lash line. Flesh-coloured eyeshadow, brushed on to your browbone, will open your eyes. If your eyes are very round,

apply a natural (not black) kohl pencil around the whole eye; if they are very narrow or almond-shaped, open them with the brow-bone/shadow trick and/or pencil the outer corner.

Plucking your eyebrows will make the whole eye area seem larger. Do not go mad, as thin eyebrows look awful, but just clean up the area beneath the arch by plucking out hairs that are not part of the main brow; the difference will be startling.

MATT OR SHIMMER?
Make-up comes in a choice of matt or shimmer finishes, and although younger faces can usually get away with most looks there are some textural guidelines for different ages. All skins – especially older ones – benefit from light, hydrating, or slightly shimmering (non-matt) bases; matt foundations can make some skins look very flat and dry, but they work well for Afro and Asian skins.

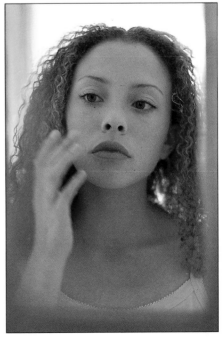

Modern foundations are able to ease out skin tone and improve imperfections in the texture of your skin.

Skin around the eyes ages quickly, so keep eye make-up very muted. Ideal colours for defining the eyes of older women include greys and soft browns; pale pinks and mauves work well as eyeshadows, with peaches and corals on cheeks and lips.

Older women should avoid shimmery eyeshadows for the simple reason that the glitter falls into the lines in the skin and makes crepey skin look much worse.

NATURAL EYE DEFINITION ON PALE SKIN

For the most natural eye make-up, apply a neutral pale beige shade from your eyelids to eyebrows; dot a grey or brown eyeliner wand across the top of your eyelash line and smudge the colour dots in with a cotton bud to create a fuzzy defining line. Apply mascara, but only partly, by wiggling the mascara wand at the base of your eyelashes to cover both top and bottom. Do not stroke the brush all the way over your lashes.

ASIAN AND AFRO BEAUTY

Choose foundations that are made specifically for black skins, or they may give a grey effect to your complexion. Powder is a staple because it helps to stabilize foundation; choose a finely milled loose, translucent one. Dark skins look best made up with rich jewel-like colours. Opt for matt eyeshadows: mauves, greys and metallics suit black skins; pinks, golds, and yellow-based browns flatter Asian skins; and dusky, earthy tones such as aubergine, dark pink, and taupe suit Afro-Caribbean skins.

HOW TO STOP EYESHADOW FROM CREASING

The key is to apply colour powder to a matt base. You can buy eyelid primers that keep oiliness to a minimum, and some matt eyeshadows contain special ingredients to help the colour stay in place.

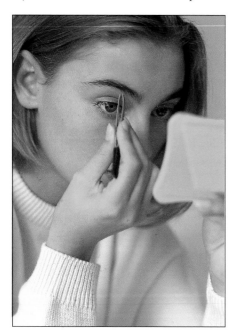

Pluck stray hairs from underneath your eyebrows to "open" the whole eye area.

Balanced use of the brighter end of the colour spectrum is very flattering to dark skins.

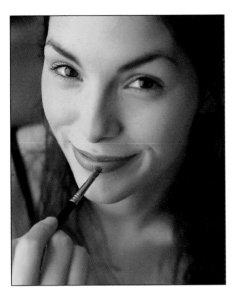

Using a fine brush to stroke on lipstick allows you to get more precise definition.

Dust loose face powder over your eyelids and then apply a thin base layer of eyeshadow colour, slowly building up the colour depth layer by layer. Using a brush makes blending easier.

COLOUR ACCURACY AND HARMONY

Test make-up shades – especially foundation – in natural light, so stand by a window or door if you can. When you are looking for a new foundation, test colours on the side of your jaw, or, if you have to, on the inside of your wrist. Avoid the back of your hand as it is a completely different colour to your face. If you cannot find exactly the right base shade, go a step lighter than your natural skin tone.

The definition of a balanced make-up is to have the perfect amount of colour on the face. No matter what age you are, too much make-up is very unflattering and can put years on you. We all love a bit of colour and most people's faces benefit from it, but try to limit the intensities to your lips or eyes, not both. If you prefer pink shades, wear a subtle, fleshy base on your eyes, and slick fuchsia on to your lips; if you like dramatic eye make-up, wear it, but keep your lips a soft (preferably neutral) colour.

CLUMP-FREE LASHES

Take time to apply your mascara: brush the first coat on one eye and then move to the other set of lashes. Then come back to the first set and apply a second coat. Clumps collect when you rush and do not let the mascara layers dry properly. If your mascara is too old, it will flake or clump because it has lost its oily mobilizing properties. Avoid pumping the wand into the dispenser as this will make the mascara dry out. Buy a new mascara every six months and make sure it is waterproof: it will stay on longer and will not smudge.

CONCEALING EVIDENCE

Concealing is a tricky task because it usually shows. To mask under-eye bags, dot the area with foundation that is slightly lighter than the one you usually wear, and don't dust powder over the top. You should use paler concealer to cover spots and scars, and always use only a tiny amount.

LIP LOOKS

Your skin tone changes from season to season so you should regularly reassess your lipstick as well as your foundation shade. Lipsticks that work best are those that have some of your skin's natural tones in their colour, such as blue-pinks or yellow-browns. A corresponding lip pencil is a valuable investment too because when you outline your lips before colouring them in, lipstick – and particularly the intense shades – will not bleed into the fine lines around your mouth.

To apply lipliner, rest the elbow of your working hand on a flat and steady surface – or on the palm of your other hand – and trace quickly and lightly around your lips; when you get near to the corners of your mouth, fade the line out by marking it more lightly. If you like, you can cover your entire mouth with lipliner: it acts as a good lipstick base. Afterwards, apply lipstick, preferably using a brush (it helps to stabilize the colour), blot the lipstick with a tissue and apply a second coat.

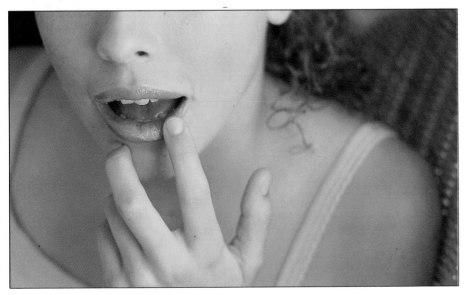

Tinted lip gloss helps to keep lips soft, and gives them a hint of sheer colour.

FIVE MINUTE MAKE-UP

You do not have to wear enormous amounts of cosmetics to be wearing proper make-up. If you do not have much time, try this routine – it is guaranteed to get you looking good in five minutes:

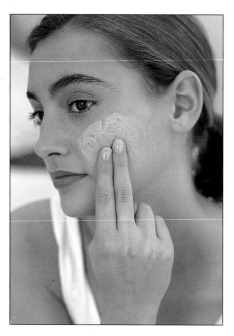

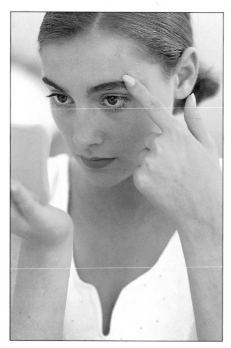

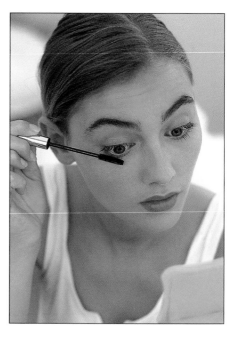

1 Apply a base of tinted moisturizer such as ordinary face cream mixed with foundation.

2 While your base settles, apply a spot of petroleum jelly to your eyebrows and then coax the hairs in your brows upwards.

3 Next, carefully brush a couple of coats of mascara on to your upper and lower lashes.

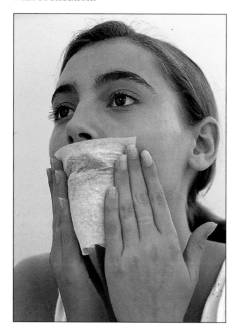

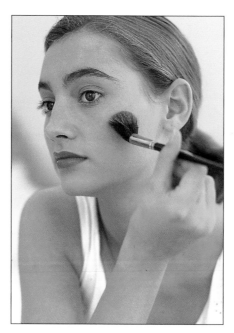

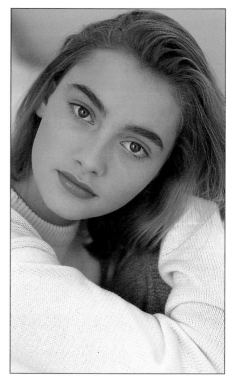

4 Apply lipstick; blot with a tissue and then apply a second coat.

5 Dust powder over your forehead, nose, lips, and chin.

DAY TO EVENING MAKE-UP – IN FIVE STEPS

Going straight out for the evening from work? Here's how to revive your make-up in five easy steps:

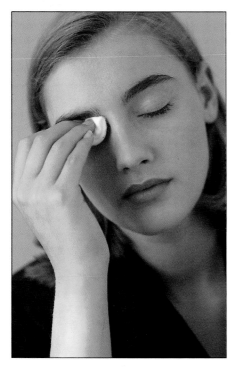

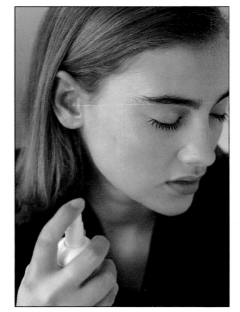

2 Check to see if your foundation needs re-touching; spritz over it with a fine spray of water and then re-powder your nose, forehead, and chin to set the make-up; dust powder over your eyelids and lips.

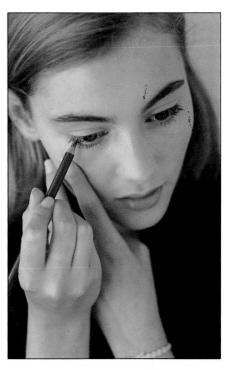

1 Remove any eye and lip make-up with oil based cleansers, taking care not to drag the skin around the eyes.

3 Re-apply eye make-up. The best evening make-up is simple: a fleshy base tone with a touch of black eyeliner over the top lid, and black mascara.

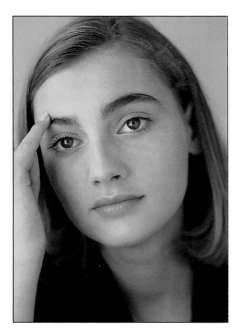

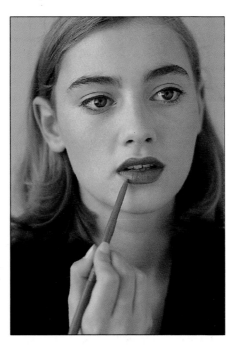

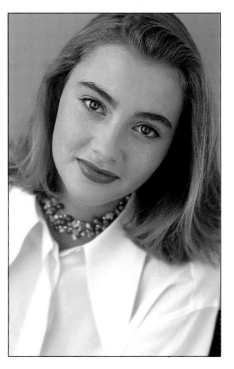

5 Re-apply lipstick: matt red is dramatic for the evening. If you prefer not to wear bright lipstick, use a slightly darker shade than the one you normally wear. Trace your lips with lipliner first; add lipstick, blot with a tissue and add a second coat.

4 Use a tiny bit of petroleum jelly to smooth your eyebrows upwards.

BEAUTY MAKEOVERS

NICKI

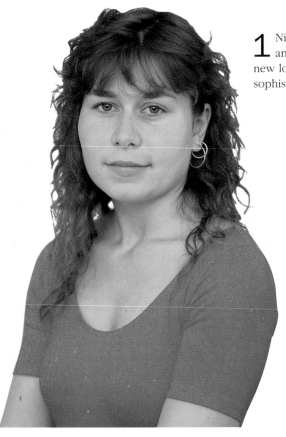

1 Nicki has dark brown hair and beige skin tones. For her new look she wants a more sophisticated style.

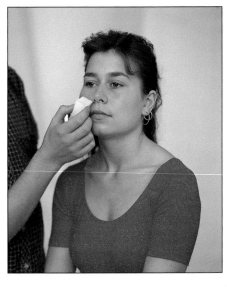

2 Paul matches colour foundation to Nicki's skin tone and applies the foundation with a cool, damp sponge onto toned, moisturised skin.

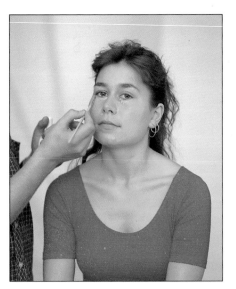

3 A dab of concealer cream – a shade lighter than the foundation – hides minor blemishes.

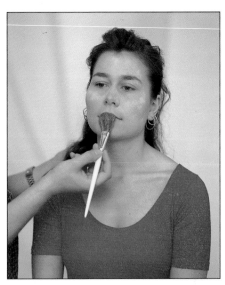

4 Beige loose powder is dusted on to Nicki's nose, chin, and forehead to set the foundation.

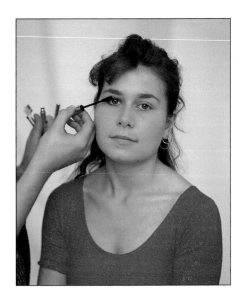

5 Paul applied a neutral beige eyeshadow to the eyelids to create a base; he added darker brown to give depth and cream to highlight Nicki's browbone and open up the eye area. A lick of dark navy eyeliner across the upper lids adds drama and enhances the blue of Nicki's eyes. Mascara completes the look.

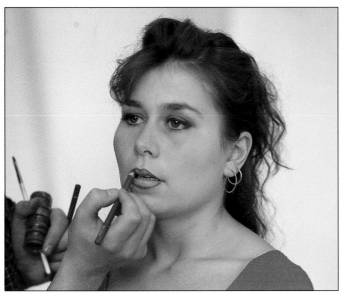

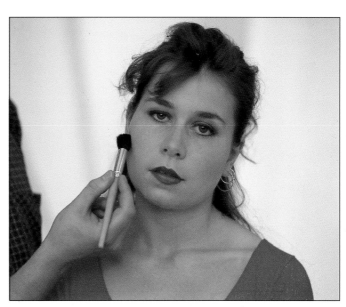

6 Lipliner is applied to outline the mouth and prepare it for lip colour. The lipstick is blotted on to a tissue; this helps to stabilize the base coat of colour.

7 Blusher, dusted on the upper cheeks, enhances the shape of Nicki's face.

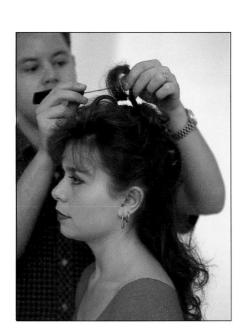

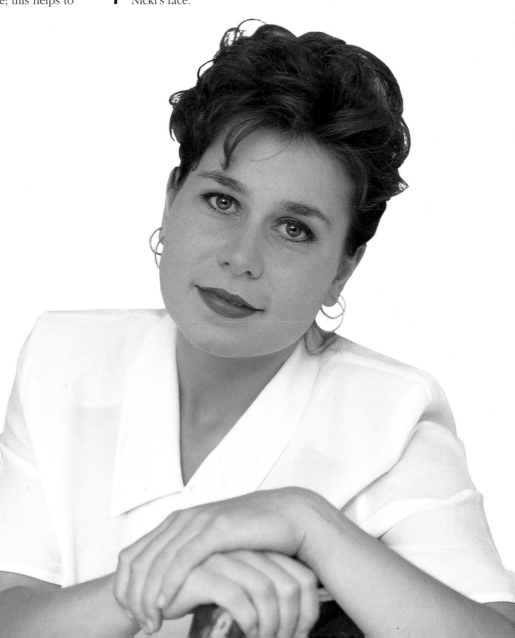

8 Paul has used Carmen rollers to give Nicki's hair body and movement. He arranges the top hair in large loops.

LUCY

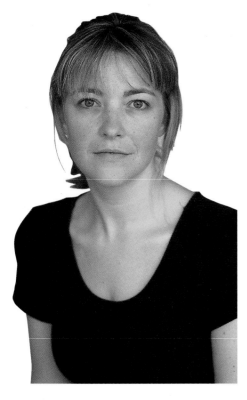

1 Lucy has a healthy outdoor look: her hair is highlighted to enhance its blonde colour and her complexion is even textured with a youthful elasticity and tone.

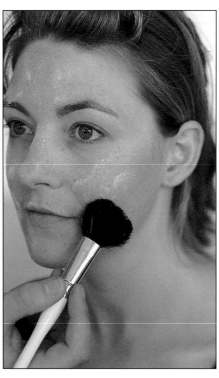

2 A very sheer foundation is used to reveal the natural beauty of Lucy's complexion.

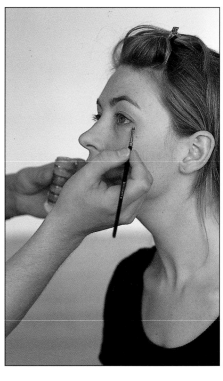

3 Paul sets the foundation with a light dusting of translucent loose powder.

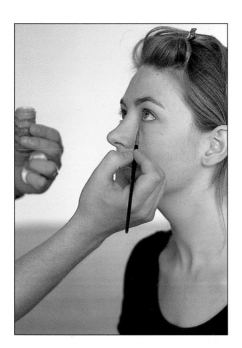

4 Shades from the earthy section of Paul's palette – taupe and a slightly deeper mushroom shade – complement Lucy's brown eyes.

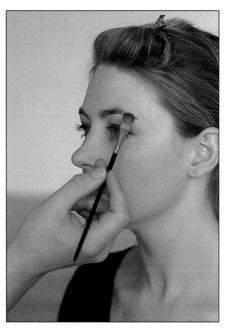

5 Paul has tweezed hairs from below the arch of Lucy's eyebrows to open up her eyes and make the area look cleaner. He uses a comb to brush the hairs upwards, another eye-opening trick.

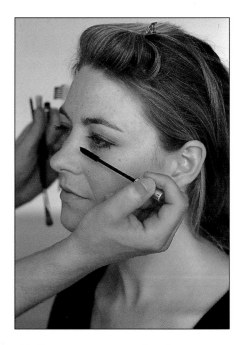

6 Brown mascara matches the eyeshadow.

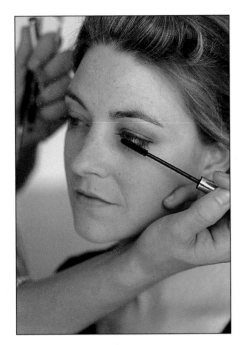

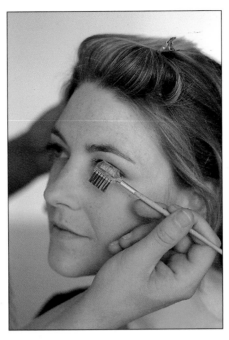

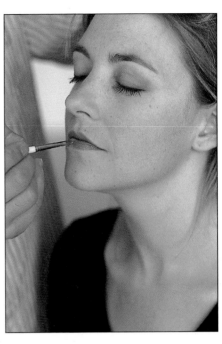

7 Mascara is applied to the lower lashes as well as the upper ones.

8 Paul combs Lucy's eyelashes with a fine-toothed comb in order to separate the lashes.

9 Lucy chooses a natural, pale pink-brown shade of lipstick.

TIP
When applying loose powder, "knead" it into your skin with the puff or a wedge of cotton wool. Remember to powder your neck as well.

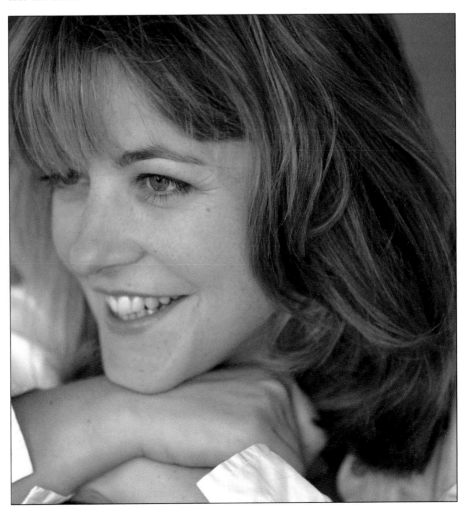

GENEVIEVE

1 Genevieve's dark colouring gives her free rein to use colours from the richer, more dramatic end of the spectrum.

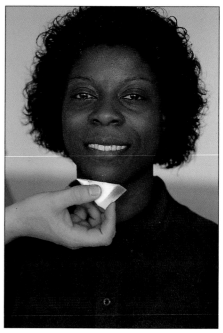

2 To combat a slightly oily complexion, Paul uses a dark beige matt foundation specially formulated for black skin so that the skin won't look chalky, but boost its clarity. Transparent loose powder is dusted over the top to set the foundation.

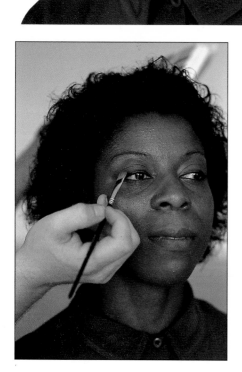

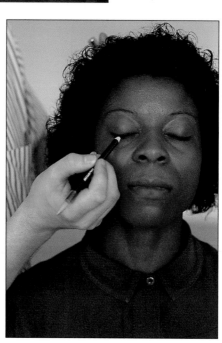

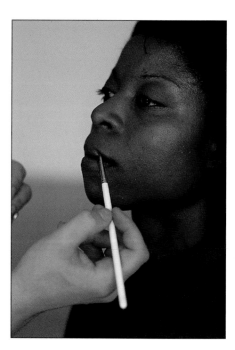

3 Paul dusts a blend of mauve eyeshadow tones on to the eyelids.

4 Black eyeliner adds drama and definition to the eyes.

5 A dark, plum-coloured lipstick complements eyeshadow and skin tones.

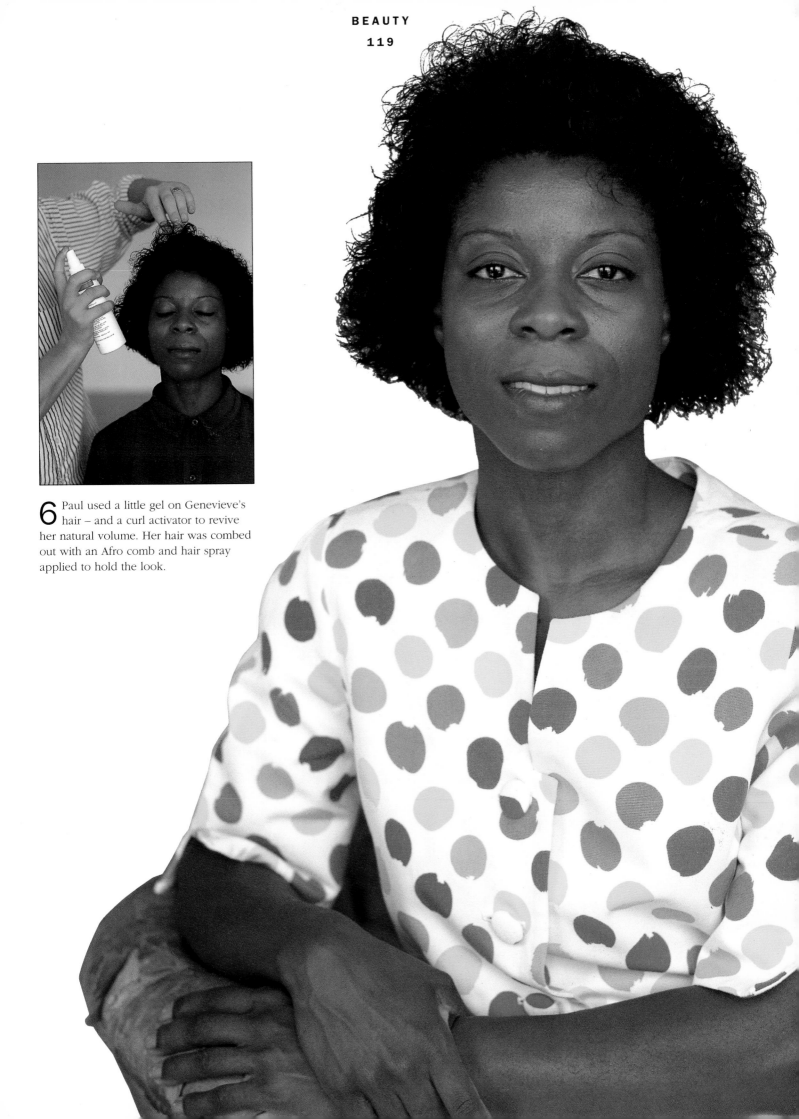

6 Paul used a little gel on Genevieve's hair – and a curl activator to revive her natural volume. Her hair was combed out with an Afro comb and hair spray applied to hold the look.

LINDA

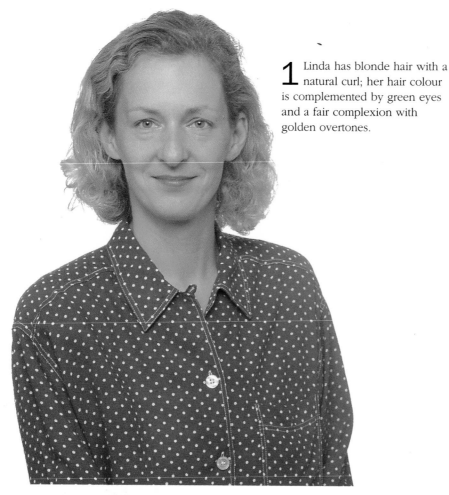

1 Linda has blonde hair with a natural curl; her hair colour is complemented by green eyes and a fair complexion with golden overtones.

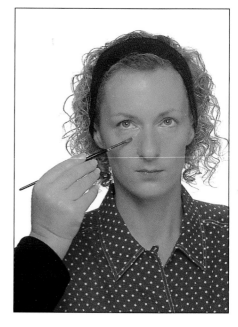

2 Bettina cleansed and moisturized Linda's skin, then dampened her hair to promote the curl. She then applied a light foundation and a slightly lighter shade of concealer under the eyes and around the curve of the nose (areas where the skin is a different tone to the rest of the face) to even out the base colour. The concealer is dotted on with a small brush and then carefully blended in.

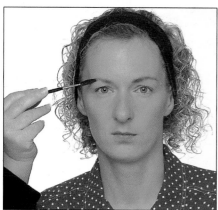

3 Very light powder is brushed over the cheekbones and under the eyes, then a translucent powder matching the foundation is applied to the rest of Linda's face. Once the powder has been brushed in, Bettina uses a small stiff brush to brush the eyebrows down so that she can see their natural shape. Using a softer brush she blends dark grey and mid brown eyeshadow, with which she darkens Linda's fair eyebrows.

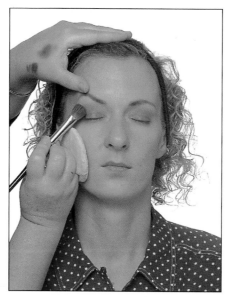

4 Eyeshadow in a neutral shade is worked over the whole eye area to provide a good base on which Bettina can build up colour over the lids in browney-grey. Eyeliner on both the top and bottom lids completes the eye make-up.

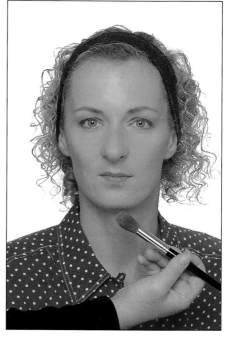

5 A taupe-coloured shadow on the end of the chin and nose contours the face.

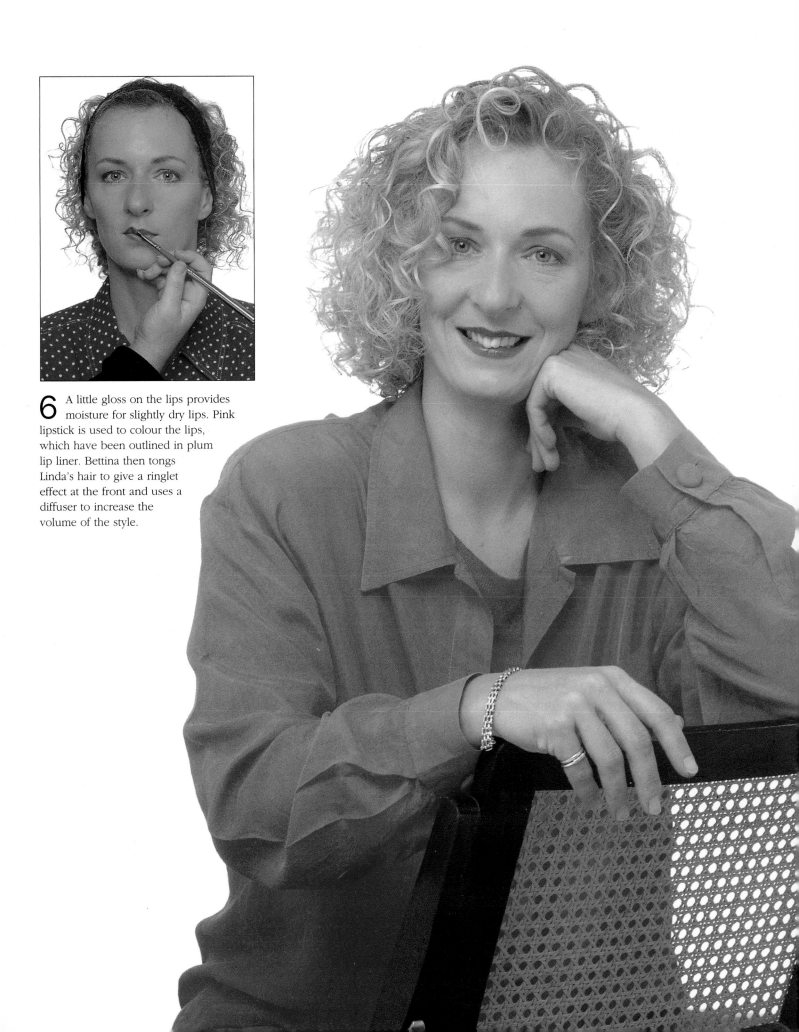

6 A little gloss on the lips provides moisture for slightly dry lips. Pink lipstick is used to colour the lips, which have been outlined in plum lip liner. Bettina then tongs Linda's hair to give a ringlet effect at the front and uses a diffuser to increase the volume of the style.

CLARE

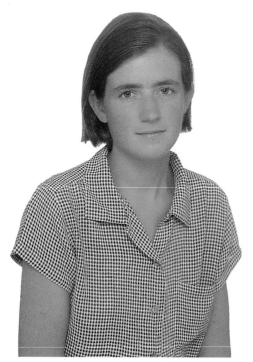

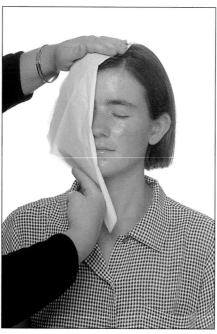

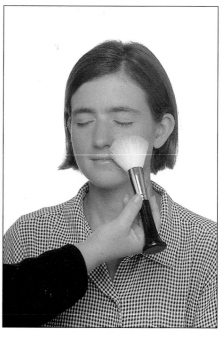

1 Clare's fresh, natural look is emphasized by pinkish tones on the cheeks.

2 Before applying foundation Bettina moistens the face with a solution of mineral water and rosewater. Using a tissue she blots the skin to remove excess moisture, leaving it just damp and more receptive to the foundation.

3 Beige lightened with ivory ensures that the high colour on the cheeks is toned down without hiding all of Clare's natural colour. Powder is applied with light, downward strokes of the brush.

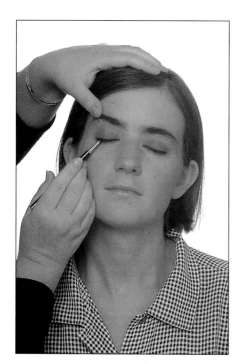

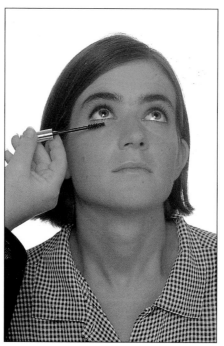

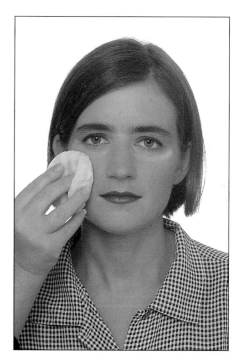

4 After covering the eyebrows with a neutral, light foundation, a blend of charcoal-grey and brown eyeshadow is used to groom Clare's eyebrows and give them a more definite shape – slightly arching and tapering off at the end.

5 Black mascara is brushed carefully on to the upper and lower lashes.

6 Clare chooses a russet-brown lipstick and blusher in a similar colour. Bettina puts white powder under the eyes to give a clean look to the eye area and emphasize Clare's eyes.

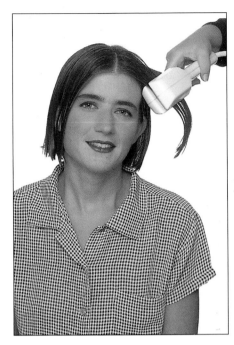

7 To complete Clare's new, modern look, hair cream is used to add shine and separation to the hair, which is then smoothed into a sleek style with a straightening iron.

TIP
When applying face powder, start at the chin and work upwards. This prevents the powder falling into the eyes from the fully-loaded brush.

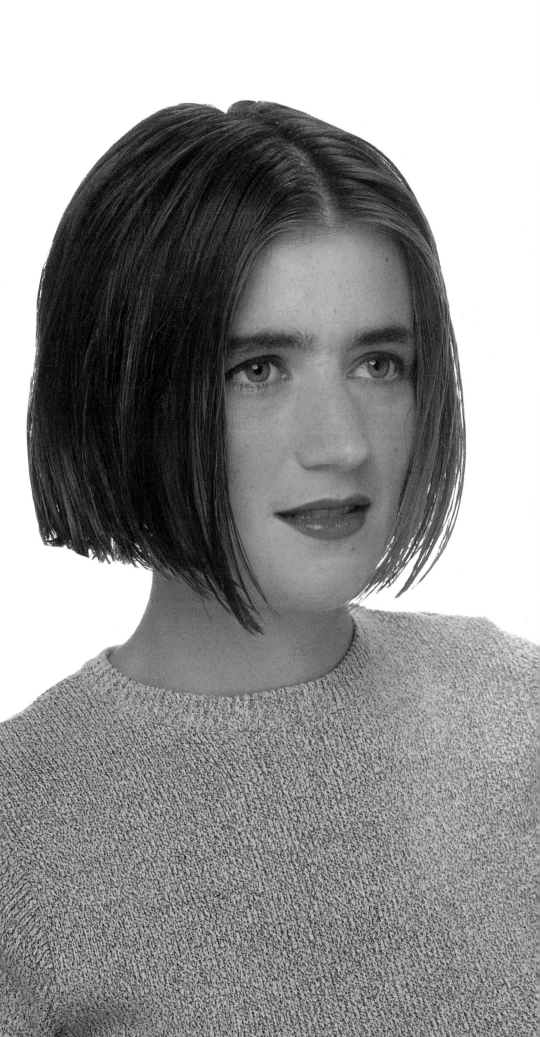

RUTH

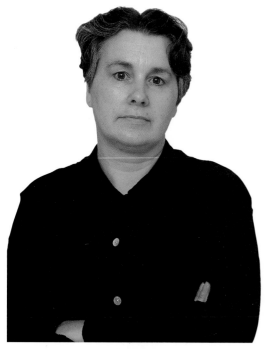

1 Ruth has good features and expressive eyes. Her black hair is tinged with silver around the temples.

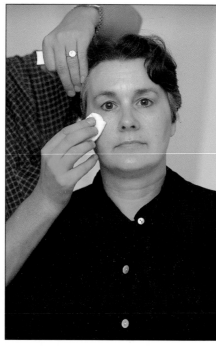

2 A light water-based moisturizing primer makes Ruth's skin matt – to help foundation last longer.

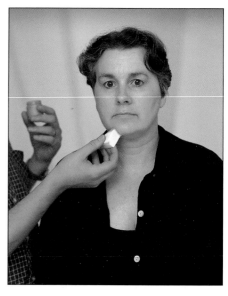

3 The primer is given time to settle before Paul "kneads" foundation over the top with a sponge.

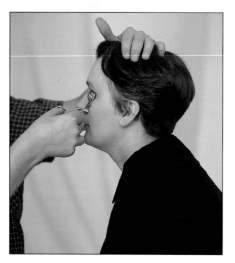

4 Eye make-up done, Paul uses conventional curling tongs on Ruth's eyelashes before sweeping mascara over the top and bottom lashes.

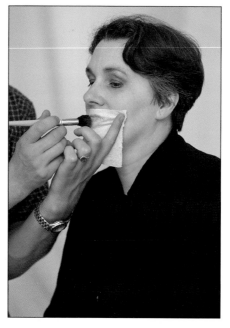

5 To stabilize the lipstick Paul blots the colour with a tissue; he then dusts loose powder on top to set it.

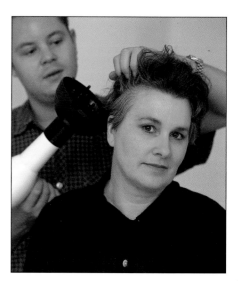

6 Paul injects maximum volume into Ruth's towel-dried hair by applying a featherlight mousse to the roots and then scrunch drying the hair with a diffuser.

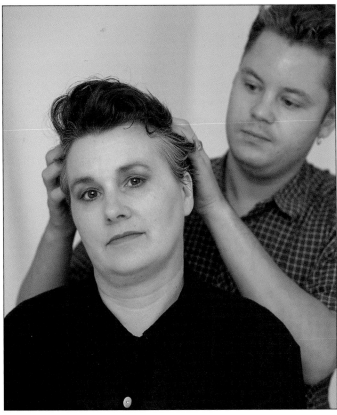

7 Paul teases Ruth's hair to a finished look with his fingers – wax adds definition to the ends.

TIP

Lipliner helps to stop lipstick from smudging or bleeding into the fine lines around your mouth. You can also use it to very slightly alter the shape and size of your lips – a trick that needs practice, otherwise you can end up looking like Tammy Faye Baker. Apply lipliner just outside the lips and you will make your mouth look bigger; trace it inside – and use a dark lipcolor, and you'll make your lips look smaller.

TIP

Experts use sponges to apply foundation for hygiene's sake; but it's more economical to use your fingers because sponges soak up a lot of foundation. Once it's on, check that there are no tidemarks around your neck and hairline in natural light.

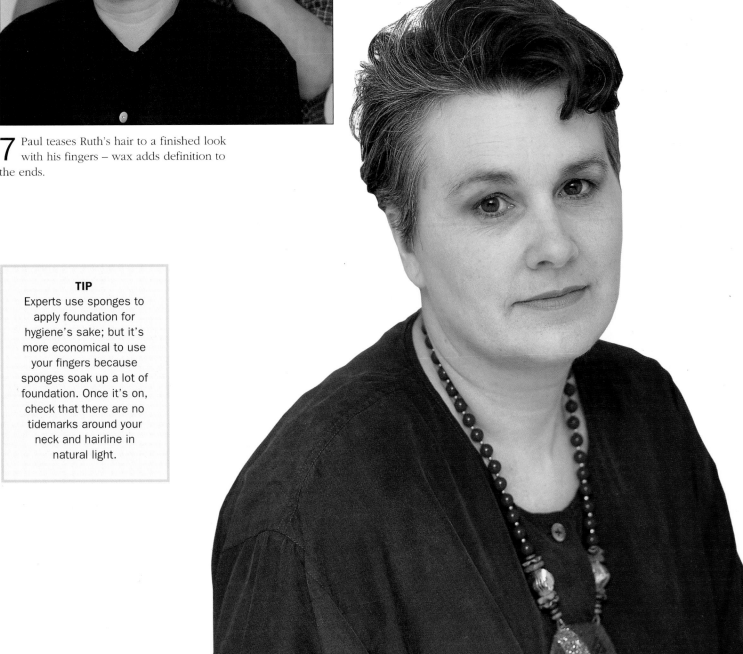

USEFUL ADDRESSES

British Nutrition Foundation
High Holborn House
52–54 High Holborn
London WC1
071-404-6504

Women's Nutritional Advisory
  Service
PO Box 268
Lewes
East Sussex, BN7 2QN

Institute for Optimum Nutrition
5 Jerdan Place
London SW6
071-385-7984

British Association of Beauty
  Therapy & Cosmetology
  (BABTAC)
Parabola House
Parabola Road
Cheltenham
Gloucestershire GL50 3HH
0242-570284

The Skin Treatment and Research
  Trust (START)
c/o Chelsea & Westminster Hospital
Fulham Road
London SW10
081-746-8000

Philip Kingsley Trichological Clinic
54 Green Street
London W1
071-629 4004

The Alternative Medicine Clinic
56 Harley House
Marylebone Road
London NW1
071-486-7490

Healthy Venues (Free central
  reservations and advisory service
  for most British health farms and
  spas) 0203-690300

Joan Price's Face Place
33 Cadogan Street
London SW3
071-589-9062

The London Esthetique
41 Queen's Gate Terrace
London SW7 5PN
071-581-3019

The International Federation of
  Aromatherapists
The Royal Masonic Hospital
Ravenscourt Park
London W6 0TN
081-846-8066

Aromaline (Advice on all aspects of
  aromatherapy)
0891-111152

Institute for Complementary
  Medicine (ICM)
PO Box 194
London SE16

Lasercare (specialize in thread vein
  removal and have branches
  throughout Britain)
1 Park View
Harrogate
North Yorkshire HG1 5LY
0423-528383

The Society of Chiropodists and
  Podiatrists
53 Welbeck Street
London W1M 7HE

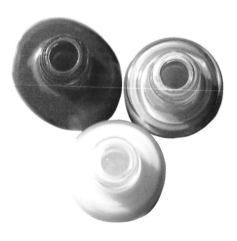

INDEX

The recipes are indexed separately and appear at the end of the general index.

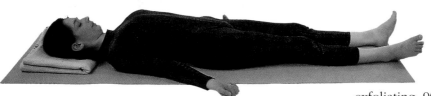

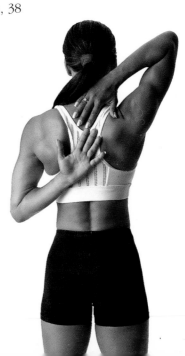

RECIPE INDEX

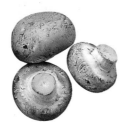

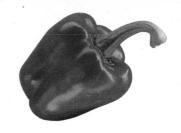

PICTURE CREDITS

Edward Allwright p59; Sue Atkinson (direction, Mira Mehta) p98; Alistair Hughes
p110 bl; Bonieventure pp120-123; Sporting Pictures (UK) Ltd pp10 bl, 11 tr, tl, 13 tr,
22 bl, br; Vyner Street Studios pp29, 50, 51, 52 tl, 53 tr, 54, 55.

AUTHOR'S ACKNOWLEDGEMENT

I would like to thank the following people for the immeasurable support they gave
me while I was writing this book: Carri Kilpatrick, Peter Clark and JJ, John Prothero,
Emma Bannister at *Options*, Anna-Marie Solowij at *Elle* and Jacki Wadeson. Grateful
thanks too to Simon and Julie Bottomley for the use of their beautiful home, Simon's
assistant Alex Forsey, and Sue at 10a Belmont Street. Finally, special thanks to my
family for knowing never to ask me how it was going but always being interested
when I felt like telling them.